LIFE STRESS
AND
ILLNESS

LIFE STRESS
AND
ILLNESS
Second Printing

Edited by

E. K. ERIC GUNDERSON, Ph.D.

Head, Epidemiology and Operational Psychiatry Division
Navy Medical Neuropsychiatric Research Unit
San Diego, California
Adjunct Professor of Psychiatry
University of California
San Diego, California

and

RICHARD H. RAHE, M.D.

Head, Biochemical Correlates Division
Navy Medical Neuropsychiatric Research Unit
San Diego, California
Adjunct Associate Professor of Psychiatry
University of California
Los Angeles, California

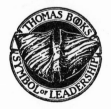

CHARLES C THOMAS • PUBLISHER
Springfield • Illinois • U.S.A.

Published and Distributed Throughout the World by
CHARLES C THOMAS • PUBLISHER
Bannerstone House
301-327 East Lawrence Avenue, Springfield, Illinois, U.S.A.

© *1974, by* CHARLES C THOMAS • PUBLISHER

ISBN 0-398-03003-0

Library of Congress Catalog Card Number: 73 14690

First Printing, 1974
Second Printing, 1979

With THOMAS BOOKS *careful attention is given to all details of manufacturing and design. It is the Publisher's desire to present books that are satisfactory as to their physical qualities and artistic possibilities and appropriate for their particular use.* THOMAS BOOKS *will be true to those laws of quality that assure a good name and good will.*

Printed in the United States of America
R-1

Government reproductions of this material may be made without charge.

Library of Congress Cataloging in Publication Data

Gunderson, Ellsworth K. Eric   1923-

Life stress and illness.

"Based upon contributions of the Symposium on Life Stress and Illness, sponsored by the Science Committee of the North Atlantic Treaty Organization (NATO) and held at Beito, Norway on June 12 to 16, 1972."

1. Medicine, Psychosomatic—Congresses. 2. Stress (Physiology)—Congresses. I. Rahe, Richard H., joint author. II. Title [DNLM: 1. Stress, Psychological—Congresses. 2. Psychosomatic medicine—Congresses. WM90 S983L 1972]
RC49.G85   616.08   73-14690
ISBN 0-398-03003-0

This book is gratefully dedicated to Captain Ransom J. Arthur, MC, USN, Commanding Officer, and to Dr. Walter L. Wilkins, Scientific Director, of the Navy Medical Neuropsychiatric Research Unit, San Diego, who have provided exceptional leadership for a wide variety of research endeavors during the past decade. They have been primarily responsible for the development of broad investigative programs in the area of life stress and illness, many of which are represented in this volume. The interdisciplinary cooperation reflected in this work, and the international recognition given to it, can be largely attributed to the wisdom and devotion to human welfare of these distinguished scientists.

CONTRIBUTORS

Captain Ransom J. Arthur, MC, USN, *Commanding Officer, Navy Medical Neuropsychiatric Research Unit, San Diego, California.*

Dr. George W. Brown, *Department of Sociology, Bedford College, London, England.*

Dr. Aubrey Kagan, *Epidemiology Unit, World Health Organization, Geneva, Switzerland.*

Dr. N. A. Kokantzis, *Department of Neurology and Psychiatry, University of Thessaloniki, Greece.*

Dr. Lennart Levi, *Director, Laboratory for Clinical Stress Research, Karolinska Sjukhuset, Stockholm, Sweden.*

Dr. E. S. Paykel, *Consultant Psychiatrist, St. George's Hospital Medical School, London, England.*

Dr. Richard H. Rahe, *Head, Biochemical Correlates Division, Navy Medical Neuropsychiatric Research Unit, San Diego, California.*

Dr. Robert T. Rubin, *Department of Psychiatry, University of California, Los Angeles, California.*

Dr. Töres Theorell, *Medical Department, Serafimerlasarettet, Stockholm, Sweden.*

Dr. Walter L. Wilkins, *Scientific Director, Navy Medical Neuropsychiatric Research Unit, San Diego, California.*

DISCUSSANTS

Dr. J. L. T. Birley, *Institute of Psychiatry, London, England.*

Dr. P. M. Brunetti, *Clinique des Maladies Mentales, Centre Psychiatrique Sainte-Anne, Paris, France.*

Dr. E. A. Haggard, *Department of Psychiatry, Abraham Lincoln School of Medicine, University of Illinois, Chicago, Illinois.*

Dr. T. J. Hunt, *Medical Research Council, Applied Psychology Unit, Cambridge, England.*

Dr. Bert King, *Organizational Effectiveness Programs, Office of Naval Research, Arlington, Virginia.*

Dr. P. D. Nelson, *Research Division, Bureau of Medicine and Surgery, Department of the Navy, Washington, D.C.*

Dr. Ranan Rimon, *Chief Psychiatrist, Finnish Armed Forces, Lahti, Finland.*

Dr. Matti Romo, *Finnish Heart Association Research Programs, Helsinki, Finland.*

Dr. W. T. Singleton, *University of Aston in Birmingham, United Kingdom.*

Dr. Gösta Tibblin, *Medical Clinik I, Sahlgrenska Sjukhuset, Göteborg, Sweden.*

PREFACE

THIS BOOK is based upon contributions to the Symposium on Life Stress and Illness sponsored by the Science Committee of the North Atlantic Treaty Organization (NATO) and held at Beito, Norway on June 12 to 16, 1972. The purpose of the symposium was to bring together investigators from several countries who were actively engaged in research on psychosocial factors in the etiology of physical and mental disease in order to assess current knowledge and evaluate future research needs.

Most of the contributors distributed their papers prior to the symposium and revised the contents on the basis of comments and discussion by participants. The final products appear as chapters in this volume and incorporate the major data and interpretations reported by the authors. The editors have attempted to bring coherence to the entire body of the text by placing the chapters in a meaningful sequence and by reducing redundancy or ambiguity in content as appropriate. However, the text remains as faithful as possible to each author's ideas and style of expression.

Drs. Romo and Tibblin as discussants presented original data of sufficient interest that the editors invited them to submit this new material as separate chapters (Chapters VI and VII). The report by Dr. Horowitz and his associates on the decline in significance of life change events over time was included as Chapter VIII because of its relevance and timeliness, even though it had not been presented at the Symposium.

The Symposium and this book were made possible by a grant from the Advisory Group on Human Factors of the NATO Science Committee. The Committee sponsors a wide range of scientific activities to facilitate communication, understanding and cooperation in the international scientific community, including conferences and symposia, advanced instruction, and cooperative research in the behavioral sciences. Dr. Richard Trumbull of the Advisory Group on Human Factors encouraged the initial proposal for the symposium, and Dr. B. A. Bayraktar of the Scientific Affairs Division, NATO, assisted greatly in the development of a viable program. The Symposium was made possible in large measure by the encouragement, guidance and support of Captain Ransom J. Arthur and Dr. Walter L. Wilkins of the Navy Medical Neuropsychiatric Research Unit, San Diego, California. The extent of their contributions to this and other scientific endeavors is reflected in the dedication of this volume. Dr. Rolf Gerhardt and his assistant, Ivar Fløistad, served as local hosts for the Symposium and greatly enhanced the work of the conference by providing pleasant and tranquil surroundings and excellent administrative arrangements.

The editors express deep appreciation for the untiring efforts of Miss Patricia Polak and Ms. Bernice Norton in the preparation of the manuscripts.

CONTENTS

ix

LIFE STRESS
AND
ILLNESS

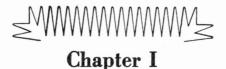

Chapter I

INTRODUCTION

E. K. ERIC GUNDERSON

IT IS OFTEN ASSUMED by physicians and laymen that ill health is somehow related to threatening or traumatic events in an individual's life. Recent distressing experiences tend to be viewed as causal or aggravating factors in the onset of health problems, and physicians regularly caution their patients to avoid upsetting situations which might hinder recovery or cause a condition to worsen. The patient's family or friends also typically advise the individual to avoid stress and tension as a means to speed recovery or avoid a recurrence. While these notions appear to be supported by casual observation and certain dramatic cases, the scientific evidence for such beliefs has been far from definitive or even consistent.

"Life stress" refers to a broad area of research concerned with events in daily living which affect susceptibility to illness; this concept in the title should not be taken to imply that this term can be precisely defined or that all potentially stressful situations can be considered. The concept merely points to a general area of emerging scientific interest which needs better operational definition and conceptual integration. The present volume hopefully advances toward this goal.

The possible deleterious effects of high rates of social change on physical and mental health have recently become an area of interest to medical and behavioral scientists. Toffler[5] popularized the notion that individuals and groups may be overwhelmed by an accelerating rate of social and cultural change in the years ahead and suffer what he calls "future shock." He defined future shock as the "distress,

3

both physical and psychological, that arises from an overload of the organism's physical adaptive systems and its decision-making processes" (p. 290). The impact of rapid social change on the health of individuals and groups is not clear, but this question offers a distinct challenge for future investigators. Rahe and his colleagues in quantifying the rate of change experienced by individuals may provide an important tool with which to address this question.

This volume presents the research findings of a number of leading investigators concerned with the effects of various life stresses on health. The Symposium on which the volume was based assembled scientists from England, Finland, France, Greece, Norway, Sweden, Switzerland and the United States, who were actively engaged in research on psychosocial stresses. The conference provided for an interchange of current research results and ideas as well as a review of major developments in the field over the past decade. The scientific program of the Symposium was organized around five major topics: concepts of social stress and disease etiology, quantitative methods for assessing life stress, precipitating factors in psychiatric illness, psychosocial factors in cardiovascular disease, and biochemical and neuroendocrine adaptations to life stress. The contents of the book have remained faithful to these topical areas, although materials presented at the Symposium have been expanded or amended in certain instances to achieve coherence and completeness.

In addition to being multidisciplinary and international in composition, the Symposium was unique in focusing for the first time on efforts to achieve quantitative scaling of life events with respect to their relative significance for future illness. Most of the studies reported are pioneering efforts, and it is recognized that much remains to be done and that it will take time to evaluate and assimilate the large amount of new information gathered in the past few years.

The many and varied uses of the term "stress" are familiar to even the casual reader in this field. At this stage of development, when approaches and terminology vary considerably, each author must delineate his own concepts and empirical methods as clearly as possible. Methodology is an important issue in several of the papers of this volume, and descriptions of experimental procedures generally are thorough. Dr. Levi firmly anchors his operational definition of the term in Selye's original conceptions of nonspecific and stereotyped physiological responses. Other authors use the term to refer to external stimulus conditions rather than responses inside the organism. Professor Singleton and Dr. Wilkins in their respective contributions to this volume comment upon some of the confusions inherent in the terms "stress" and "illness" and note certain definitions and their connotations. The problems of defining stress have been considered at length elsewhere[1, 3, 4] and will not be pursued in detail here.

Dr. Levi as Director of the Laboratory for Clinical Stress Research, Karolinska Institute, Stockholm, has made an enormous contribution to the study of psychosocial stress over the past decade. He currently is editing the proceedings of a series of symposia cosponsored by the World Health Organization titled *Society, Stress and Disease.* Volume I, *The Psychosocial Environment and Psychosomatic Diseases*, was published in 1971, and Volumes II and III are in preparation.

In the second chapter Levi defines basic terms and presents a conceptual model for viewing the interrelationships of psychosocial stress, physiological mechanisms and disease. He reviews the evidence that a variety of psychosocial stressors affect physiological processes and traces the multiple possible origins and pathways of disease development.

Dr. Kagan, who as Head of the Unit for Research in Epidemiology, World Health Organization, worked closely with Dr. Levi in formulating approaches to the analysis of psychosocial factors in disease, is particularly interested in using such knowledge to prevent illness. He suggests economical strategies for conducting the large-scale longitudinal research needed in the future and illustrates how specific hypotheses might be tested utilizing Levi's conceptual model and experimental epidemiological methods.

Chapters IX and X present full accounts of the important work by Dr. Paykel and Dr. Brown on precipitating factors in psychiatric illness. Using sophisticated methodologies, these investigators have produced the most definitive results extant linking recent life events and depressive or schizophrenic illness. Following the pioneering work of Holmes and Rahe,[2] they too have applied quantitative scaling methods to determine the most crucial family and social experiences in the onset of severe psychiatric illness.

The series of papers by Rahe and his associates on life change measures and their relationships to cardiovascular and other disease reflects the extensive collaboration that has existed among Finnish, Norwegian, Swedish and United States investigators over the past few years. Following Dr. Rahe's outline of the development of life change scales and their application to large naval populations for predicting both minor and major illnesses, a number of specific studies are reported which yielded substantive findings concerning life changes and onset of disease in Finland, Norway, Sweden and the United States, or significant developments in life event scaling and scoring methods. Dr. Nelson, in his comments on Dr. Rahe's paper, discusses the need for advanced multivariate methods of analysis because of the complexities of person-environment transactions and the multiple factors that influence health over extended periods of time.

Dr. Rubin provides an overview of research on severe psychological stress in humans and describes biochemical and neuroendocrine response patterns under extremely stressful training conditions. Military life offers special opportunities to study adaptation to hostile or unusual environments, and Dr. Rubin and others have taken advantage of these situations to study biochemical and psychological responses to severe stress under field conditions.

Captain Ransom Arthur, Commanding Officer of the Navy Medical Neuropsychiatric Research Unit, San Diego, describes psychological and medical consequences of extreme stress and deprivation in concentration camp inmates and views the historical context of prisoner of war treatment in the two World Wars, the Korean War and the Vietnam War. Dr. Arthur is currently responsible for the medical research program that is an integral part of rehabilitative measures designed to ameliorate the adverse effects of long confinement among recently released American prisoners of North Vietnam.

The importance of cultural differences in determining the origins and intensities of psychosocial stress is indicated in the paper by Dr. Kokantzis and his colleagues. This delineation of stressful factors in Greek society is a vivid illustration of the cultural specificity of certain psychosocial pressures and conflicts.

Dr. Wilkins, Scientific Director of the Navy Medical Neuropsychiatric Research Unit, gives a thoughtful summary of the issues discussed at the Symposium and some suggestions for enlarging our conceptual framework. He considers the problems of definition, particularly the ambiguities of the acute-chronic continuum in disease, and surveys the many social and biological factors that influence health.

REFERENCES

1. Appley, M.H., and Trumbull, R.: *Psychological Stress*. New York, Appleton-Century-Crofts, 1967.
2. Holmes, T.H., and Rahe, R.H.: The social readjustment rating scale. *J Psychosom Res, 11*:213-218, 1967.
3. Levine, S., and Scotch, N.A.: *Social Stress*. Chicago, Aldine, 1970.
4. McGrath, J.E. (Ed.): *Social and Psychological Factors in Stress*. New York, Holt, Rinehart and Winston, 1970.
5. Toffler, A.: *Future Shock*. New York, Random House, 1970.

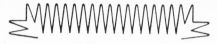

Chapter II

PSYCHOSOCIAL STRESS AND DISEASE: A CONCEPTUAL MODEL

LENNART LEVI

OBJECTIVES

THE EVIDENCE that environmental *physical* stimuli may cause physical disease—in the sense that exposure to or avoidance of such stimuli increases or decreases the chance of becoming ill or reverses ill health when it occurs—is established for a large number of environmental factors and diseases.

The role of extrinsic psychosocial stimuli is not so clear. In presenting a survey of present knowledge, we shall consider some hypotheses, speculations and research concerning the relationships between psychosocial stimuli and (1) mechanisms thought to be associated with disease, (2) precursors of disease and (3) disease itself.

In this chapter an attempt will be made to focus on the general *non*specific aspects of man's reaction to a variety of psychosocial stimuli. The author is clearly aware of the theoretical and clinical importance of the stimulus as well as of response *specificity* but feels that the nonspecific aspects are not only equally important but have so far attracted less attention.

DEFINITIONS

First we shall define the terms that represent the basic elements of our conceptual model.[31]

1. *Psychosocial stimuli.* In this context we are referring to stimuli which originate in social relationships or arrangements (i.e. in the environment), affect the organism through the mediation of higher

8

nervous processes, and may be suspected, under certain circumstances and in certain individuals, of causing disease.

2. *Psychobiological program.* This is propensity to react in accordance with a certain pattern, e.g. when solving a problem or adapting to an environment. Determinants of this program in an organism are genetic factors and earlier environmental influences.

3. *Mechanisms.* These are physiological reactions in the organism induced by psychosocial stimuli which, under some conditions of intensity, frequency or duration, and in the presence or absence of certain interacting variables, may lead to precursors of disease, and, eventually, to disease itself.

Stress is used here in the sense that Selye[59, 60] described it, namely the nonspecific response of the body to any demand made upon it; a stereotyped, phylogenetically old adaptation pattern, primarily preparing the organism for physical activity, e.g. fight or flight. These Stone Age responses, which may be provoked by a variety of psychosocial and other conditions of modern life, when no physical action is possible or socially acceptable, have been suspected of eliciting physical and mental distress or malfunction, or even structural damage. Briefly, then, stress is one of the *mechanisms* under certain circumstances suspected of leading to disease.

4. *Precursors of disease.* These are malfunctions in mental or physical systems which have not resulted in disability but which, if continued, will do so.

5. *Disease.* Disease is disability caused by mental or somatic malfunction. Disability is failure in performance of a task. This must always include tasks considered essential, might include tasks considered normal, and, when more is known, will include tasks that are considered optimal. (In applying this definition it is necessary to state the level of the biological hierarchy to which it refers. Disease as defined is different at the cell, organ and organism level.)

6. *Interacting variables.* These are intrinsic or extrinsic factors, mental or physical, which alter the action of "causative" factors at the mechanism, precursor or disease stage. By "alter" we mean they promote or prevent the process that might lead to disease.

Examples to clarify the use of these terms will be given below. It must be said now that although it is often possible to categorize factors according to the above definitions, there are many occasions when the category is not clear or when categories are interchangeable. Nevertheless, we think they will facilitate discussion, and probably lead to a better understanding of the problem.[5, 31]

A CONCEPTUAL MODEL FOR PSYCHOSOCIALLY MEDIATED DISEASE AND SOME HYPOTHESES

The combined effect of psychosocial stimuli (1) and the psychobiological program (2) determines the psychological and physiological reactions (mechanisms (3), for example, stress) of each individual. These may, under certain circumstances lead to precursors of disease (4) and to disease itself (5). This sequence of events can be promoted or counteracted by interacting variables (6). The sequence is not a one-way process but constitutes part of a cybernetic system with continuous feedback. Our conceptual model[6, 33, 62] of the above-mentioned relationships in the pathway of psychosocially mediated disease has been presented in Figure II-1.

Our experimental work has been based on this model and on the following series of hypotheses. Every psychosocial change can act as a stressor in Selye's sense of the word. In response to such an exposure, and in accordance with the phylogenetically old adaptation pattern ("psychobiological program," *cf.* Fig. II-1) which man has

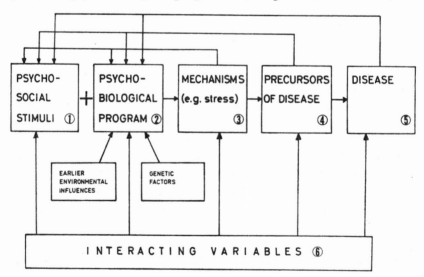

Figure II-1. A conceptual model for psychosocially mediated disease (Figure from Levi[38]).

in common with his prehistoric ancestors and with all primates, the neuroendocrine system becomes activated, preparing the organism for physical activity, e.g. fight or flight, even in situations where such reactions are clearly inadequate. The resulting increase in "stress (Selye)" may lead to an "increased rate of wear and tear" in the organism, and in predisposed individuals eventually lead to disease of one type or another.

Should this be so, one might expect (a) that a great variety of stimuli, physical as well as psychosocial, would, directly or indirectly,[43] evoke physiological responses, some features of which (e.g. changes in sympathoadrenomedullary activity and possibly in plasma lipid level) are stereotyped and nonspecific, (b) that a positive and statistically significant relationship should exist between the degree of life change[53] and sympathoadrenomedullary activity (as reflected in adrenaline excretion) and between life change and various types of morbidity, and (c) that hyperlipoproteinemia should predict not only death in degenerative myocardial disease but also death in general, being a mechanism, a predictor and/or precursor in a nonspecifically evoked pathogenetic process. Evidence supporting these hypotheses would point to the existence of a common, general, nonspecific factor in the pathogenic process, in addition to a number of more or less specific ones.

One of the crucial points in this chain of reasoning is that "stress (Selye)" can be evoked by every or almost every change, including psychosocial change. This would mean that increases in "stress (Selye)" should occur as concomitants not only of psychological reactions usually described as unpleasant but also of those described as clearly pleasurable. If this is so, not only the unpleasant reactions but the pleasant ones too should be accompanied by "an increased rate of wear and tear in the organism." This aspect of psychophysiological relationships has been almost totally neglected in the past.

Over the past few decades the concept of stress has become increasingly popular and is now often used by many behavioral scientists and by laymen to indicate a sequence of events that almost by definition is regarded as annoying, distressful, and/or noxious and harmful. This is not the way the term is used here. True, Selye and others usually assume that "stress (Selye)" is positively related to "the rate of wear and tear in the organism," thus being potentially harmful at least from the viewpoint of an internist. However, one should not forget that "stress (Selye)" or certain aspects of it may very well be beneficial from, say, the *performance* viewpoint, particularly when the performance involves physical activity. As to psychological performance, an inverted-U relationship has often been demonstrated between efficiency and arousal level (*cf.* O'Hanlon[50] and Frankenhaeuser[19]). In a long series of studies, Frankenhaeuser and her group have shown that high adrenaline excretors usually perform significantly better in tasks involving perceptual conflict, choice-reaction and under-stimulation, but not in those involving over-stimulation, where the opposite is the case.

TYPE OF EVIDENCE TO BE REVIEWED

The relationships shown diagramatically in Figure II-1 have been studied in several kinds of investigation, in animals and in man.

In neurophysiological studies, different parts of the brain have been stimulated chemically or electrically and concurrent psychic and physiologic reactions have been measured to clarify pathogenic mechanisms.[1,48] In studies making use of psychological, sociological and epidemiological methods, groups of patients and matched control groups of healthy subjects have been compared for recent or premorbid exposure to various psychosocial stimuli, or with respect to "program" or interacting variables. Studies have been prospective or retroprospective. They show associations between psychosocial stimuli or interacting variables and mechanisms, between mechanisms and precursors of disease, and between psychosocial stimuli and disease. Attempts have also been made to assess the relative importance of genetic and environmental factors in the pathogenic process by comparing uniovular and biovular twins who were subjected to different environmental influences after birth. Studies have also been made of the entire pathogenic process as represented in Figure II-1, subjects or groups with certain characteristics being exposed to psychosocial stimuli assumed to be noxious, and the reactions in terms of mechanisms, precursors and disease being studied over time. Studies with precursors and *diseases* as endpoints have been made on animals, and analogies have been made with respect to corresponding processes in man. Generally, two classes of psychosocial stimuli have been applied: the specific and the nonspecific.[69]

The *specific* stimuli have little or no effect in themselves and assume significance only because of their capacity to act as signals and symbols. The nature and degree of the psychological and physiological reactions they evoke are dependent mainly on individual past experience. Symbols that are gravely threatening to a certain individual may be meaningless to a neutral observer, and vice versa.

The other approach involves *nonspecific* stimuli, which influence the mechanisms in almost every subject whatever his past experiences, although the degree of the reaction may vary considerably from individual to individual.

In both cases, the responses are markedly modified by a great number of interacting variables. Some of these variables have been experimentally manipulated.

Some of these studies will be referred to below as evidence of a relationship between psychosocial stimuli, interacting variables, mechanisms, precursors of disease and disease. Where possible we will indicate whether this relationship is certain, probable or speculative.

PSYCHOSOCIAL STIMULI AND PHYSIOLOGICAL MECHANISMS

Some General Considerations

First we will discuss some of the psychosocial *stimuli* that have been suspected to be pathogenic, under certain circumstances and in certain individuals.

As mentioned above, every psychosocial (or physical) environmental change can evoke "stress (Selye)." A perusal of the literature leaves the reader with the impression that the relationship between psychosocial stimulation and "stress (Selye)" can be best described as a U-shaped curve, *cf.* Figure II-2. The highest stress levels are usually found at the extremes of the stimulation continuum, i.e. during the exposure to over- or under-stimulation. In general, deprivation or excess of almost any influence is found to be stress provoking in Selye's sense of the word. For instance, high stress levels may be induced during sensory deprivation and sensory overload, in response to extreme affluence as well as to extreme poverty, parental over-protection as well as parental deprivation, extreme permissiveness as well as extreme restriction of action, etc.[5, 30, 31]

In an impressive series of studies, Rahe[53] has demonstrated the pathogenic significance of the degree of life change, although his

Life Stress and Illness

"STRESS (SELYE)"

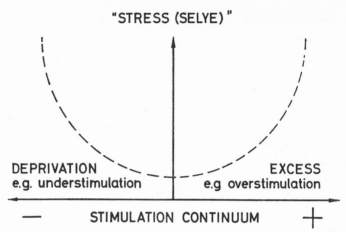

Figure II-2. Relation between physiological stress and level of stimulation. (Fig. 1:3 from Levi.[6]).

studies did not cover the mechanisms involved. Rahe's model of the relationship between life change (the sum of pleasant and unpleasant changes) and morbidity seems to be unipolar, i.e. the higher the life change, the greater the risk for subsequent morbidity. One is tempted to consider whether the model shown in Figure II-2 is applicable to Rahe's general hypothesis too. If so, life change could be just another example of stimulation, which would mean that very low as well as very high degrees of life change would be accompanied by high levels of "stress (Selye)."

Examples of experimental psychosocial stimuli will be given later in the present chapter. Suffice it to emphasize that many of the stimuli are not "purely" psychosocial and that very often the experimental or "real life" condition exposed the subject to a rather complex mixture of stimuli, which makes it extremely difficult indeed to demonstrate that a certain reaction, precursor or disease is causally related to this or that specific psychosocial stimulus.

In his penetrating discussion of the *nonspecificity* concept in stress theory, Mason[43] further emphasizes the difficulties implied in all attempts to partial out the primary effects of purely physical stimuli (e.g. cold, heat, physical trauma, physical exertion) from the secondary effects elicited by *psychological reactions* to them. At least with reference to adrenocortical function, he puts forward the alternative hypothesis that the nonspecificity and stress concepts should be regarded not as physiological but rather as behavioral, i.e. involving a higher level of central nervous system function than was previously realized. Although it would have been tempting to carry this discussion further, it does not fall directly within the scope of the present discourse (which is centered on the responses to psychosocial stimuli only) and will therefore not be dealt with in more detail.

The *mechanisms* demonstrated to be influenced by such psychosocial stimuli can be classified into the following rather broad categories: (1) mental (higher nervous) processes, (2) endocrine processes, especially hypophyseal, adrenal and thyroid function, (3) lymphatic and immunoreactive processes, and (4) other physiological processes.

In the present context we will focus on the *endocrine* mechanisms, particularly on the secretion of adrenaline, noradrenaline, corticosteroids and thyroxine. Although there probably are many other endocrine mechanisms, these have been considered particularly relevant and studied most.

Sympathoadrenomedullary Activity

It is well established that the sympathoadrenomedullary system is influenced by a great variety of psychosocial stimuli in animals as well as in man.[59] It has been claimed that if a sympathoadrenomedullary stimulation lasts too long or is repeated too often, the result will first be functional disturbances in various organs and organ systems.[11] It has further been hypothesized that such a dysfunction, if long-standing and/or intense, may result in permanent structural changes of pathogenic significance at least in predisposed individuals.[49, 52, 67] The theory that the sympathoadrenomedullary system reacts by an increased secretion of adrenaline in various emergency states, including those elicited by psychosocial stimuli, was put forward by Cannon and summarized by him as early as 1929. Twenty-five years passed, however, before this increased secretion was actually demonstrated.

In 1954, using Euler's new, sensitive, fluorimetric methods, Euler and Lundberg[17] first demonstrated an increased urinary catecholamine excretion in air force pilots and passengers during ordinary flight, and they attributed this to the psychosocial stimuli arising from the situation to which the subjects were exposed. In 1957 and 1958, Elmadjian, Hoagland and their collaborators at the Worchester

Foundation published data demonstrating an enhanced urinary catecholamine excretion in professional hockey players as well as in amateur boxers and psychiatric patients in situations comprising a variety and combination of psychosocial and physical stimuli.[12] Using a composite program of emotionally charged films, a stimulus that can be considered to be rather "purely" psychosocial, Euler et al.[15] demonstrated that this type of stimulus was equally effective in evoking such catecholamine reactions.

Since then, enhanced sympathoadrenomedullary activity has been demonstrated in response to a wide variety of situations comprising psychosocial stimuli[38] and a variety of laboratory situations characterized by over-stimulation, under-stimulation, anticipation and conflict.[19]

These studies clearly imply exposure to psychosocial (several of them also to physical) stimuli. However, some of these exposures have been of relatively short duration, while others clearly do not belong to the everyday experience of an ordinary population.

However, a number of the stimuli used in studies at our laboratory[20] do relate closely to habitual activity and some have been of prolonged duration. In *laboratory* studies, groups of subjects have been exposed to a variety of psychosocial stimuli including: (a) simulated industrial work (sorting of steel balls), (b) simulated office work (proofreading), (c) appearance before an audience, (d) film programs chosen to induce anxiety, aggressiveness, and other emotional reactions, (e) simulated psychomotor tasks, and (f) prolonged function under simulated ground combat conditions. In a series of *field* studies, the reactions of various occupational groups to real life stimuli have been studied, namely, the stimuli arising from the subjects' own work situation. These situations included those facing (a) telephone operators, (b) invoicing clerks and IBM operators paid a salary, (c) the same subjects paid on a piece-work basis, (d) office clerks subjected to changes in work environment (conventional offices and office landscapes, and different noise levels), (e) supermarket cashier girls (during rush hours and ordinary conditions), (f) paper mill workers working in three shifts, night and day, and (g) engine drivers working irregular shifts at various seasons.

Further data indicating an increased liberation of catecholamines in response to variety of psychosocial stimuli or in different states of emotional arousal have been presented in detail elsewhere[38] and clearly indicated that psychosocial stimuli do, indeed, influence sympathoadrenomedullary activity.

Adrenocortical Activity

Increased adrenal cortical activity has been noted in response to many threatening life situations[38] whereas viewing Disney naturestudy films actually lowered the 17-hydroxycorticosteroids in plasma.[24]

For review in the field of psychosocial stimuli and adrenal cortical response see Hamburg,[22] Berkun et al.,[2] Rubin and Mandell[58] and Mason.[39] Briefly, it is generally agreed that adrenal cortical stimulation occurs in response to a variety of psychosocial stimuli, but that the hypophyseoadrenocortical system reacts more slowly and requires somewhat higher stimulus intensities before reaction than does the hypothalamoadrenomedullary system. A comprehensive discussion of the reactions of the hypophyseoadrenocortical system is to be found in Yates and Maran.[70]

Thyroid Activity

The evidence concerning the relationship between psychosocial stimuli and thyroid function is less conclusive. Stimulation of the anterior hypothalamus or median eminence as well as of the hippocampal formation produces a definite increase in thyroid hormone secretion, as does stimulation of the cervical sympathetic nerve and the vagal nerve.[45] According to Rees and Moll,[55] the hypothalamus is involved in the maintenance of the secretion rate of thyroid stimulating hormone (TSH) under normal conditions, possibly through the mediation of a thyrotropin-releasing factor.[46] A long-acting thyroid stimulator (LATS), probably of pathogenic significance in Grave's disease, has also been reported.[26, 44, 46] Recently, Persky et al.[15] reported a statistically significant relationship between LATS and Thematic Apperception Test (TAT) and Holtzman test hostility content as well as between emotional arousal and TSH.

A variety of hormones, the catecholamines probably being the most potent and physiologically important, have been reported to influence thyroid function. Thus, adrenaline injection in man has been reported to raise TSH and protein-bound iodine (PBI) levels, without, however, altering iodine uptake;[29] on the other hand, Reiss et al.[56] report an increased uptake, with a maximum three to four hours after the injection. As with the related problem of stressor effects on thyroid function, part of the controversy is probably explained by the tendency to apply results obtained in animal experiments to considerations of thyroid physiology in man; furthermore, there is a time and a dose dependency of catecholamine-provoked thyroid reaction in that small doses probably increase and larger doses inhibit thyroid secretion, *cf.* Soderberg[63] and Ramey.[54]

As mentioned previously, it has been found that emotional reactions due to psychosocial stimuli are accompanied by a marked increase in adrenal cortical and medullary activity in humans, *cf.* Levi.[36] Most conspicuously, there is a rise in catecholamine excretion, sometimes to levels indicative of phaeochromocytoma. It is conceivable that these endogenous catecholamines affect thyroid function in much the same way as do exogenous catecholamines, and, if so, one or more links in the hypothalamic-hypophyseal-thyroidal chain are used as a target area.

Against this background, many studies have been made in which animals have been exposed to various environmental stimuli. The results are diverse and conflicting. This may be due, at least in part, to (a) differences preceding stimulus exposure, (b) specific effects of the various stimulus procedures applied, and (c) reactions specific to the species of mammals used in the experiments, in addition to the more obvious factors of (d) assay methods, (e) variations in attempts to control extraneous influences like dietary and nondietary iodine intake, and (f) criteria of thyroid function.

Exposure of sheep to insertion of a cannula into the jugular vein has been reported[18] to produce rapid but transient rises in plasma protein-bound iodine (PBI) and [131]PBI. Subsequently, after these changes had subsided, similar rises were demonstrable after a series of firework explosions, and, most consistently, after exposure to a barking dog. These rises lasted up to two hours. The same authors reported that restraint was followed by an increase in [131]PBI, but after training no such effect was observed.

As to previous studies in man, a number have attempted to relate different psychiatric clinical states[9, 23, 41, 46, 40] and fluctuations in these states to the thyroid function of the patients in question. Thus, Board et al.[3] reported PBI levels distinctly higher than in controls in thirty patients within twenty-four hours of their admission to the psychiatric section of a general hospital. Similarly, Hetzel et al.[27] reported increases in serum PBI in euthyroid patients subjected to stressful real-life experiences. Related results have been reported by Kleinsorge et al.[32]

Wolff[68] described fluctuations in plasma protein-bound iodine in association with exposure to stressful life experiences. Increases of as much as 100 percent were recorded in some subjects. Some changes took place within an hour of the beginning of the stimulus exposure, a psychiatric interview. In a similar investigation, Tingley et al.[66] examined the protein-bound iodine on control days as well as on stress days (exams for the medical student subjects) and found significant increases during the latter conditions. Similarly, three out of four medical students, exposed to an important examination, reacted with a significant elevation of thyroidal [132]I uptake.[7] More recently, Persky et al.[51] and Dewhurst et al.[10] have reported a statistically significant relationship between emotional reactions of various kinds and TSH levels. Exposing a total of sixty-three army officers and corporals to a seventy-five-hour vigil including seventy-two hours of intellectual performance and/or performance in an electronic shooting range under controlled environmental conditions, Johansson et al.[28] demonstrated a highly significant increase in protein-bound iodine, in individual cases to levels clearly above what are usually considered normal limits. This study is reported in detail by Levi.[38] Briefly, then, it may be concluded that a variety of psychosocial stimuli may elicit significant increases in protein-bound iodine as well as in other indices of thyroxine release in animals as well as in man.

Psychosocial Stimuli: Influence on Human Physiology

Thus, there is good evidence for a variety of effects of psychosocial stimuli on neuroendocrine function. The neuroendocrine reactions thus elicited can, theoretically, in turn influence all or nearly all existing physiological variables.

The thyroid hormones have been shown to increase the turnover of carbohydrates, lipids, calcium and magnesium, the heart rate and contractility, and total peripheral resistance, the secretion of hydrocortisone and growth hormone, and the sensitivity of some tissues to the catecholamines. The catecholamines are powerful vasoactive agents with pronounced effects on carbohydrate and lipid metabolism. The adrenal cortical hormones regulate, among other things, the carbohydrate metabolism and the metabolism of minerals and water. Consequently, a very large number of physiological processes are influenced, directly or indirectly.

In summary, we know that psychosocial stimuli cause physiological changes, which in turn *could* lead to precursors and disease.

INTERACTION VARIABLES, PRECURSORS AND DISEASE

Interacting variables may be predisposing or protective. Either may be extrinsic (environmental) or intrinsic. Many predisposing interacting variables that appear to be physical in nature may have a psychical element, e.g. heat, noise, overcrowding, malnutrition (*cf.* Mason[43]). Many of the protective interacting variables are of a psychosocial origin, e.g. habituation, adaptation, coping and substitution. Partly depending upon the presence, or absence, of such interacting variables, psychosocial stimuli may or may not influence physiological mechanisms, precursors or even disease itself.

Some of the psychosocially evoked changes in physiological function do in turn evoke proprioceptive signals to the cerebral cortex. In some individuals, and under certain circumstances, even perfectly "normal" signals of this type may be interpreted by the individual as symptoms of disease (as in the case of hypochondriasis). If the psychosocial stimulation exemplified above is pronounced, prolonged or often repeated, and/or if the organism is predisposed to react because of the presence of predisposing or absence of protective interacting variables, the results may be hyper-, hypo- or dysfunction in one or more organs and organ systems. Examples of such reactions are tachycardia and palpitations, vasovagal syncope, pain of vasomotor or muscular origin, hyperventilation, increased or decreased gastrointestinal peristalsis, etc. These reactions may, but need not, be accompanied by unpleasant emotional reactions such as anxiety, depression, apprehension, etc.

It is often postulated that the development of psychosocially induced diseases is preceded by a "precursor" state characterized by malfunction of mental and physiological systems without apparent disability.

However, as mentioned in connection with the definitions, it is sometimes impossible to demarcate the mechanisms from the precursors or from disease itself. This is particularly so when, in clinical practice, the mechanism and, more often, the precursor, is given the disease label, e.g. as in the case of *gastrointestinal distress*. Thus, there is no sharp borderline between "normal" reactions on the one hand and hypochondriacal reactions and psychological and/or physiological dysfunction characterized as precursors or diseases on the other. Besides, the definition of the level where normality ends and disease begins is closely interrelated with the social psychology of labeling.[42] Evidence concerning the reactions described above has been reviewed elsewhere.[4, 8, 11, 21, 34, 37, 57, 61, 64, 65, 67]

Further, psychosocial stimuli may also influence health by impeding recovery and aggravating disability, whatever the etiology of the primary disease. Such a psychosocially induced response may be rooted, for example, in an intense anxiety over the disease or the situation, and possibly complicated by secondary gains such as utilization of the disease as a means of avoiding responsibility, justifying one's incapacity and providing a release from social pressure.

The precursors and diseases mentioned above are all clearly influenced by psychosocial stimuli. They are all characterized by disturbed function of one type or another, but presumably not by more or less chronic functional or even structural changes. The role of pyschosocial stimuli in the etiology and pathogenesis of "psychosomatic diseases" where such changes have taken place (as in the case of peptic ulcer, bronchial asthma, essential hypertension, thryotoxicosis, and degenerative heart disease) is less clear, partly because so little is known about the etiology and pathogenesis of these disorders.

According to some of the hypotheses mentioned above, the human organism's pattern of response to a variety of environmental stimuli, including the psychosocial ones, constitutes a phylogenetically old adaptational process ("stress" in Selye's sense), preparing the organism for physical activity, usually for fight or flight. However purposeful these activities may have been in the dawn of the history of mankind, they have ceased to be very adequate in the adaptation of modern man to the endless number of socioeconomic changes, social and psychological conflicts, and threats involved in living in a highly industrialized modern, urban society. Furthermore for social reasons, man has to repress many of his emotional outlets and motor activities. This creates a situation in which there might very well be a disintegration between the expression of emotion, the neuroendocrine con-

comitants of emotion and the psychomotor activities likely to accompany such emotion. For example, in a marital or occupational
setting, modern man may feel anxiety or aggression and exhibit the
neuroendocrine concomitants of the emotional reaction without
showing it in his facial expression or verbal or gross motor behavior.
On the other hand, situations do occur when man is compelled to
exhibit emotional expressions and to perform physically or verbally
in a way grossly incongruous with his actual neuroendocrine and
emotional state. If this "stress" pattern of response to psychosocial
stimuli and/or this psychophysiological discrepancy lasts long
enough, it has been suspected to be of pathogenic significance. Indeed, processes of this kind have been claimed to constitute a major
factor in the etiology of several diseases in the field of internal medicine. An early notice of this psychosomatic relationship is to be
found in Ecclesiastes 30:24 (about 200 B.C.), indicating that "envy
and wrath shorten the life."

The evidence for and against this and related hypotheses comes
primarily from animal experiments, epidemiological studies, and
physiological measurements and observations in clinical practice. A
detailed presentation and discussion of such data fall outside the scope
of this chapter. In this context, it may suffice to recall the proposed
relation between psychosocial stimuli and catecholamines, plasma
lipids, corticosteroids, thyroid function and electrolytes, and to mention the relationship between catecholamines, hyperlipidemia and
atherosclerosis, and the combined action of catecholamines, corticosteroids, thyroid hormones and potassium deficiency in degenerative
heart disease.

PSYCHOSOMATIC RESEARCH
Some General Considerations

"Scientific study of emotion and of the bodily changes that accompany diverse emotional experience marks a new era in medicine.
We know now that many physiological processes which are of pro-
found significance for health . . . can be controlled by way of emotions. In this knowledge we have the key to many problems of prevention and treatment of illness." This was written some thirty-five
years ago, by Flanders Dunbar, in the introduction of her first large
survey of experimental and clinical studies in the field of "emotions
and bodily changes." However, in spite of the innumerable studies

published since, part of which have been reviewed above, this "key to many problems of prevention and treatment" has been elusive, and we are still confronted with a confusing variety of controversial *data* on psychosomatic relationships, not to mention the interpretations of and the hypotheses built on these data.[42]

A perusal of the literature in this field, however, leaves the reader with a feeling that part of this controversy might have been avoided (a) by more attention being paid to methodological problems and (b) by subjecting the various links in the hypothetical chain of events mentioned above (Fig. II-1) to a more systematic and comprehensive study. Here, we review previous knowledge and suggest some new ways of examining Mason's key question,[42] "What normal body mechanisms are involved in psychosomatic illnesses and how and why do they go wrong?"

Psychosomatic research is primarily concerned with physiological and psychological reactions induced by environmental stimuli that are usually referred to as "psychosocial." In most of the psychosomatically oriented medical literature, various disorders have been related to a number of such stimuli to which the patients usually are said to have been exposed prior to and/or in conjunction with the onset of the particular disease.[35].

The constellations of these stimuli inherent in everyday life—at work, in the family, even in the clinical situation—are, however, usually very complex and the interaction with physical stimuli of many types complicates the picture still more. It is, therefore, very difficult clinically or even epidemiologically to distinguish between the various links in the hypothetical chain of events and to map out the relative importance, if any, of one or another of the many psychosocial influences.[47]

As a complement to clinical and epidemiological studies, researchers in various disciplines and parts of the world have increasingly made use of psychophysiological and psychoendocrine experiments by exposing an individual or a group to various *stimuli*, single or combined, intense or moderate, of long or short duration, etc. Or a stimulus has been applied to various *individuals* or *groups*—patients and healthy controls, females and males, young and old, extroverts and introverts, people who do or do not make use of various coping mechanisms, etc. In either case, we may want to study psychological and/or physiological functions at various levels of complexity, using different methods of measurement and different "languages" in describing the reactions and their underlying mechanisms. Theoretically, we would like to study the entire sequence of events in all relevant groups when exposed to all relevant stimuli, the measurements comprising all relevant variables. This, of course, is not possible. Therefore, in medical research, we are likely to concentrate on stimuli and mechanisms suspected by some as potentially of pathogenic significance, or on individuals or groups likely to be more (or less) at risk than the general population.

The Stimuli

The use of different kinds of functional and provocation tests has long been practiced in physiology and clinical medicine, the patient being exposed to such stimuli as physical work, ACTH, insulin, cold and allergens, in order to test the quality and quantity of his response. The psychophysiological experiment makes use of psychosocial stimuli in a corresponding way, by exposing subjects to (a) threats to self-esteem or physical integrity, (b) various types of high or low sensory input, (c) open-ended situations or (d) environmental change in general, of varying magnitude, frequency and/or velocity.

As already mentioned, these stimuli may be specific, i.e. have a special meaning for the subject, or *nonspecific*, that is to say active to some extent on all individuals irrespective of the subject's genetically and environmentally determined psychobiological "programming."[69]

In a review of psychophysiological stress studies, Harris et al.[25] classified experiments of this type according to the kind and duration of stimulus employed. According to these authors, short-term stimuli may be exemplified by and categorized into: (1) failure stressors (e.g. subjects told about previous failures but given one more chance to solve insoluble problems), (2) workload, pacing and distraction stressors (e.g. subjects have to perform a task, sometimes at above-normal speed, sometimes being distracted by meaningful or meaningless noises, flashing lights, electric shocks, etc.) and (3) fear-inducing stressors (real or simulated threats of criticism, of being fired, of physical danger, or unpredictability implied in the stimulus situation, etc.).

Long-term stimuli are similarly subdivided into four categories: (1) combat stressors (subjects are exposed to attack situations or a defensive stand over long periods of time), (2) stressors of hazardous duty (e.g. of submarine and aircraft personnel, or soldiers near the front line area but not in actual battle), (3) stressors of confinement and isolation (e.g. submarine or astronaut duty, prison confinement, low sensory input) and (4) prolonged performance stressors (vigilance tests, monotonous work, etc., resulting in fatigue).

Most of the short-term studies have been performed in psychological or physiological laboratories, whereas the long-term stressors are often given in a real-life setting. Many of the laboratory studies have been well designed scientifically but may lack realism and meaning to the subjects tested. The real-life situations, on the other hand, usually have been realistic enough but in many cases badly controlled, and so their results are indecisive.

Interacting Variables

It is common knowledge that different individuals do not react identically to any given stimulus or set of stimuli. Neither does an individual react identically on various occasions even if we try to keep the stimulus conditions reasonably constant. The reasons for this inter- and intra-individual variability are manifold—processes like habituation, adaptation, learning and coping, constitutional factors, genetic as well as acquired group interaction, interaction effects with other stimuli, just to mention a few. Factors like these must be taken into account when choosing our subjects and the circumstances for their study.

Reactions

On the reaction side, a study of "emotions and bodily changes" usually implies simultaneous determination of these two sets of variables and an analysis of the relation between them, if any. Trying this, we face a series of problems. Needless to say, the actual, subjective experiences of our subjects are not accessible to direct measurement, neither are the basic neuroendocrine processes which are closely linked to these experiences. We have to be content with indirect studies of these phenomena, e.g. the subject's verbal report of his experiences, or measurements of hormone levels in body fluids.

A very large number of such psychological and physiological variables have been described and measured in man's response to various psychosocial stimuli. Psychological responses have been measured by direct observation, by interviews, questionnaires and projective techniques. A great number of physiological measurements have dealt with various aspects of cardiovascular, respiratory, gastrointestinal and renal function, each study usually focusing on a few variables, and without paying much attention to the underlying physiological mechanisms, treating them as a "physiological black box."[42]

What To Measure and Why

Another set of studies—including those by the present author—have dealt not so much with specific organ functions but with the more basic, integrative aspects of physiological response, i.e. the neuroendocrine reactions. During the last two decades, chromatographic, isotope, immunoassay, microspectrophotometric and fluorimetric methods of measurement have become available that allow a relatively detailed study of functions related to what is commonly called the hypophyseoadrenocortical and hypothalamicoadrenomedullary axes. In man, these functions have usually been studied by determining various hormones (and compounds, influenced by these hormones) in blood, urine, liquor and in various tissues.

In some of these studies, the psychological responses were assessed simultaneously, with respect to self-ratings by the subjects, and to performance when work of one type or another was involved.

The primary target for the studies conducted at our laboratory has been the human organism's sympathoadrenomedullary activity measured as urinary excretion of adrenaline and noradrenaline, analyzed fluorimetrically.[16] This set of variables was chosen for several reasons. First the responses of the sympathoadrenomedullary system have been studied less than those of the adrenocortical system, partly because satisfactory methods for assay of hormones belonging to the last-named system have been available for a longer period of time. Second, it is known that the catecholamines may play important roles in the physiology of the human organism, in health as well as in disease. Third, earlier studies conducted by the present author and by others gave reason to suspect a rather close relationship between sympathoadrenomedullary and psychological function.

Some of the studies comprised measurements of other physiological variables as well (e.g. plasma lipids, erythrocyte sedimentation rate, serum iron, protein-bound iodine, urine flow and specific gravity, urinary creatinine, ECG pattern), to provide data relevant to specific objectives of the study.[38]

GENERAL OBJECTIVES OF OUR STUDIES

Investigations from our laboratory all had the following general objectives in mind.

Firstly, to ascertain whether, and, if so, to what extent exposure to some psychosocial stimuli encountered by modern man (e.g. piecework) actually elicits significant changes in sympathoadrenomedullary and other physiological functions as reflected in changes in a number of blood and urine constituents. Should this be so, it may turn out to be necessary to take the psychosocial situation of the patient into account when clinically interpreting laboratory data on these constituents.

Secondly, to find out whether any physiological reactions provoked in this way have a reasonably high and steady correlation with the subjective state experienced and, one may hope, reported by the subject. The objective would be to see if the physiological reactions could be used as a predictor or index of subjective reactions in cases where these are not readily accessible to direct measurement with psychological methods,[13, 14] as an index which cannot be masked by verbal or overt behavior.[42]

Thirdly, to study possible interindividual differences in the "programming" of the organism as reflected in differences in different groups' (males and females) reactions to identical stimuli.

Fourthly, to see if physiological reactions to psychosocial stimuli experienced under relatively long-term conditions were similar to those produced in acute laboratory experiments.

Fifthly, to identify mechanisms by which psychosocial stimuli are likely to lead to disease.

Much of the discussion to be presented in the following chapters is based on the "stress (Selye)" concept. As repeatedly emphasized by Selye, this concept should be regarded as a working hypothesis, to be evaluated and re-evaluated with refined methods. The use of this concept does not necessarily imply an unconditional acceptance of an *absolute* "nonspecificity." Clearly, there is a progressively greater burden of proof involved as we move through the sequence of hypotheses that a particular bodily response is evoked (a) in a relatively great diversity of situations, to (b) by a relatively great diversity of stimuli, to (c) by "*every* stimulus." At the present stage, all of these hypotheses seem to deserve evaluation.

THE "STRESS (SELYE)" CONCEPT

As demonstrated in a number of investigations in our laboratory, psychosocial stimuli do clearly influence urinary catecholamine excretion, either enhancing or lowering it, depending on the stimuli and on the psychophysiological starting position of the organism. Enhancement occurs not only in response to stimuli which most subjects rate as predominantly "unpleasant" but also when the self-ratings indicate predominantly "pleasant" emotional reactions in most of the subjects. We interpret these data as supporting the hypothesis concerning "stress (Selye)" as the nonspecificity (or stereotypy) of physiological reaction to a variety of stimuli, taking into account not only "unpleasant" reactions but "pleasant" ones as well. Probably it is the intensity, and not the quality of these reactions which is the main correlate of "stress (Selye)." Our results further support the assumption that sympathoadrenomedullary activity constitutes part of "stress (Selye)."

Of course, this is not meant to imply that no specific relationship exists between psychosocial stimuli and physiological response, or between subjective response and physiological concomitants. On the other hand, our findings do not support hypotheses proposed by other authors concerning a specific relationship between, for example, anxiety and adrenaline excretion or between aggression and noradrenaline excretion. This interpretation is in agreement with findings reported by Frankenhaeuser and her group.[19]

True, the "stress (Selye)" nonspecificity in physiological response discussed so far relates exclusively to *psychosocial* stimuli. On the other hand, it is well-known that a considerable number of *physical* environmental stimuli do evoke a similar response, *inter alia* involving sympathoadrenomedullary activity.

As indicated previously, there can be several *degrees* of nonspecificity in bodily response, the same reactions occurring in response to (a) relatively great diversity of *situations*, (b) a relatively great diversity of *stimuli* (physical and/or psychosocial) and (c) *every* stimulus. Our results do not allow any definite statement as to which of these alternatives is most valid, but they do contribute to illustrate the nonspecificity postulated by Selye and emphasize the need for further research in this field.

REFERENCES

1. Bajusz, E., and Jasmin, G.: *Major Problems in Neuroendocrinology.* Basel, S. Karger, 1964.
2. Berkun, M.M., Bialek, H.M., Kern, R.P., and Yagi, K.: Experimental studies of psychological stress in man. *Psychol Monogr, 76* (15), 1962.
3. Board, F., Persky, H., and Hamburg, D.A.: Psychological stress and endocrine functions. *Psychosom Med, 18*:324, 1956.
4. Bykov, K.M.: *The Cerebral Cortex and the Internal Organs.* Moscow, Foreign Languages Publishing House, 1959.
5. Carlestam, G., and Levi, L.: Urban conglomerates as psychosocial human stressors: general aspects, Swedish trends, and psychological and medical implications. A contribution to the U.N. Conference on the Human Environment, Stockholm. Royal Swedish Ministry for Foreign Affairs, 1971.
6. Chapanis, A.: Men, machines and models. In Marx, M.H. (Ed.): *Theories in Contemporary Psychology.* New York, Macmillan Co., 1964, p. 104.
7. Crooks, J., quoted by Dewhurst, K.E., El Kabir, D.J., Harris, G.W., and Mandelbrote, B.M.: A review of the effect of stress on the activity of the central nervous-pituitary-thyroid axis in animals and men. *Confin Neurol, 30*:171, 1968.
8. Delius, L., and Fahrenberg, J.: *Psychovegetative Syndrome.* Stuttgart, Georg Thieme Verlag, 1966.
9. Dewhurst, K.E., El Kabir, D.J., Exley, D., Harris, G.W., and Mandelbrote, B.M.: Blood levels of the thyrotropic hormone, protein-bound iodine, and cortisol in schizophrenia and affective states. *Lancet,* 2:1160-1162, 1968.
10. ———, El Kabir, D.J., Harris, G.W., and Mandelbrote, B.M.: A review of the effect of stress on the activity of the central nervous-pituitary-thyroid axis in animals and man. *Confin Neurol, 30*:171, 1968.
11. Dunbar, F.: *Emotions and Bodily Changes.* New York, Columbia University Press, 1954.
12. Elmadjian, F.: Excretion and metabolism of epinephrine and norepinephrine in various emotional states. Lima, Peru, *Proc of the 5th Pan Amer Congr of Endocrinology,* 1963, p. 341.
13. Euler, U.S. v.: Quantitation of stress by catecholamine analysis. *Clin Pharmacol Ther, 5*:398, 1964.
14. ———: Evaluation of stress by quantitative hormone studies. Internat Symposium on Man in Space, Paris, 1962. Wien, Springer-Verlag, 1965, pp. 308-326.

15. ————, Gemzell, C.A., Levi, L., and Strom, G.: Cortical and medullary adrenal activity in emotional stress. *Acta Endocrinol (Kbh)*, 30:567, 1959.

16. ————, and Lishajko, F.: Improved technique for the fluorimetric estimation of cathecholamines. *Acta Physiol Scand*, 51:348, 1961.

17. ————, and Lundberg, U.: Effect of flying on the epinephrine excretion in Air Force personnel. *J Appl Physiol*, 6:551, 1954.

18. Falconer, J.R., and Hetzel, B.S.: Effect of emotional stress and TSH on thyroid vein hormone level in sheep with exteriorized thyroids. *Endocrinology*, 75:42, 1964.

19. Frankenhaeuser, M.: Experimental approaches to the study of human behaviour as related to neuroendocrine functions. In Levi, L. (Ed.): *Society, Stress and Disease: The Psychosocial Environment and Psychosomatic Diseases.* London, Oxford University Press, 1971, pp. 22-35.

20. Froberg, J., Karlsson, C.-G., Levi, L., and Lidberg, L.: Physiological and biochemical stress reactions induced by psychosocial stimuli. In Levi, L. (Ed.): *Society, Stress and Disease: The Psychosocial Environment and Psychosomatic Diseases.* London, Oxford University Press, 1971, pp. 280-295.

21. Gellhorn, E., and Loofbourrow, G.M.: *Emotions and Emotional Disorders.* New York, Harper & Row, 1963.

22. Hamburg, D.A.: Plasma and urinary corticosteroid levels in naturally occurring psychological stresses. In Korey, Saul R. (Ed.): *Ultrastructure and Metabolism of the Nervous System.* Baltimore, Williams and Wilkins, 1962.

23. Hamburg, D.A., and Lunde, D.T.: Relation of behavioural, genetic, and neuroendocrine factors to thyroid function. In Spuhler, J.N. (Ed.): *Genetic Diversity and Human Behavior.* Chicago, Aldine Publishing Co., 1967, pp. 135-170.

24. Handlon, J.H., Wadeson, R.W., Fishman, J.R., Sachar, E.H., Hamburg, D.A., and Mason, J.W.: Psychological factors lowering plasma 17-hydroxy-corticosteroid concentration. *Psychosom Med*, 24:535, 1962.

25. Harris, W., Mackie, R.R., and Wilson, C.L.: Performance under stress. Technical Report VI. Los Angeles, Human Factors Research, 1956.

26. Hetzel, B.S.: The aetiology and pathogenesis of hyperthyroidism. *Postgrad Med J*, 44:363, 1968.

27. ————, Schottstaedt, W.W., Grace, W.J., and Wolff, H.G.: Changes in urinary nitrogen and electrolyte excretion during stressful life experiences, and their relation to thyroid function. *J Psychosom Res*, 1:177, 1956.

28. Johansson, S., Levi, L., and Lindstedt, S.: Stress and the thyroid gland: A review of clinical and experimental studies, and a report of own

studies on experimentally induced PBI reactions in man. Report 17. Stockholm, Lab for Clin Stress Res, 1970.

29. Johnston, I.D.A.: The effect of surgical operation on thyroid function. *Proc R Soc Med, 58*:1017, 1965.

30. Kagan, A.R., and Levi, L.: Adaptation of the psychosocial environment to man's abilities and needs. In Levi, L. (Ed.): *Society, Stress and Disease: The Psychosocial Environment and Psychosomatic Diseases.* London, Oxford University Press, 1971, pp. 399-404.

31. Kagan, A.R., and Levi, L.: Health and environment—psychosocial stimuli. A review. Report 27. Stockholm, Lab for Clin Stress Res, 1971. *Man, Science and Medicine,* in press.

32. Kleinsorge, G., Klumbies, H.-J., Bauer, C.B., Dressler, E., Finck, W., and Wolkner, E.: *Angina Pectoris, Angst und Schilddrusenfunktion.* Jena, Fischer, 1962, pp. 40-43.

33. Lachman, R.: The model in theory construction. In Marx, M.H. (Ed.): *Theories in Contemporary Psychology.* New York, Macmillan Co., 1964, p. 78.

34. Lader, M.H. (Ed.): Studies of anxiety. *Br J Psychiatr,* Spec Pub No. 3. Ashford, Kent, Headley Brothers, 1969.

35. Levi, L. (Ed.): Emotional stress and military implications. Stockholm, Forsvarsmedicin 3, Supplement 3, 1967. (Simultaneously published by Karger, S., Basel-New York, and by American Elsevier, New York, 1967.)

36. ————: Sympatho-adrenomedullary and related biochemical reactions during experimentally induced emotional stress. In Michael, R.P. (Ed.): *Endocrinology and Human Behaviour.* London, Oxford University Press, 1968.

37. ————: *Society, Stress and Disease: The Psychosocial Environment and Psychosomatic Diseases.* London, Oxford University Press, 1971.

38. ————: Stress and distress in response to psychosocial stimuli. *Acta Med Scand, 191,* Supplement 528, 1972. (Simultaneously published in book form by Pergamon Press, Oxford, 1972.)

39. Mason, J.W.: A review of psychoendocrine research on the pituitary-adrenal cortical system. *Psychosom Med, 30*:576, 1968.

40. ————: A review of psychoendocrine research on the sympathetic-adrenal medullary system. *Psychosom Med, 30*:631, 1968.

41. ————: A review of psychoendocrine research on the pituitary-thyroid system. *Psychosom Med, 30*:666, 1968.

42. ————: Strategy in psychosomatic research. *Psychosom Med, 32*:427, 1970.

43. ————: A re-evaluation of the concept of "non-specificity" in stress theory. *J Psychiatr Res, 8*:323, 1971.

44. McKenzie, J.M.: The thyroid-activating hormones and hypothalamic control. In Levine, R. (Ed.): *Endocrines and the Central Nervous System.* Baltimore, Williams and Wilkins Co., 1966, pp. 47-58.

45. ————, and Solomon, S.H.; Neuroendocrine factors in thyroid disease. In Bajusz, E., and Jasmin, G. (Eds.): *Major Problems in Neuroendocrinology*. Basel, S. Karger, 1964, pp. 312-327.

46. ————, and Solomon, S.H.: Neuroendocrine factors in thyroid disease. In Bajusz, E. (Ed.): *An Introduction to Clinical Neuroendocrinology*. Baltimore, Williams and Wilkins Co., 1967, pp. 320-324.

47. Mechanic, D.: Problems and prospects in psychiatric epidemiology. In Hare, E.H., and King, J.K. (Eds.): *Psychiatric Epidemiology*. London, Oxford University Press, 1970.

48. Nalbandov, A.V. (Ed.): *Advances in Neuroendocrinology*. Urbana, Illinois, University of Illinois Press, 1963.

49. Nodine, J.H., and Moyer, J.H. (Eds.): *Psychosomatic Medicine: The First Hahnemann Symposium*. Philadelphia, Lea and Febiger, 1962.

50. O'Hanlon, J. F.; Vigilance, the plasma catecholamines, and related biochemical and physiological variables. Technical Report 782-2. Goleta, Calif.: Human Factors Research, 1970.

51. Persky, H., Zuckerman, M., and Gurtis, G.C.: Endocrine function in emotionally disturbed and normal men. *J Nerv Ment Dis, 146*:488, 1968.

52. Raab, W. (Ed.): *Preventive Cardiology*. Springfield, Ill., Thomas, 1966.

53. Rahe, R.H.: Life crisis and health change. In May, P.R.A., and Wittenborn, J.R. (Eds.): *Psychiatric Drug Responses: Advances in Prediction*. Springfield, Ill., Thomas, 1969.

54. Ramey, E.R.: Relation of the thyroid to the autonomic nervous system. In Levine, R. (Ed.): *Endocrines and the Central Nervous System*. Baltimore, William and Wilkins Co., 1966, pp. 309-324.

55. Rees, G.P. van, and Moll, J.: Influence on thyroidectomy with and without thyroxine treatment on thyrotropin secretion in gonadectomized rats with anterior hypothalamic lesions. *Neuroendocrinology, 3*:115, 1968.

56. Reiss, R.S., Forsham, P.H., and Thorn, G. W.: Studies on the interrelationship of adrenal and thyroid function. *J Clin Endocrinol, 9*:659, 1949.

57. Roessler, R., and Greenfield, N.S. (Eds.): *Physiological Correlates of Psychological Disorder*. Madison, Wisc., The University of Wisconsin Press, 1962.

58. Rubin, R.T., and Mandell, A.J.: Adrenal cortical activity in pathological emotional states: A review. *Am J Psychiatr, 123*:387, 1966.

59. Selye, H.: The concept of stress in experimental physiology. In Tanner, J.M. (Ed.): *Stress and Psychiatric Disorder*. Oxford, Blackwell, 1960.

60. ————: The evolution of the stress concept—stress and cardiovascular disease. In Levi, L. (Ed.): *Society, Stress and Disease: The Psychosocial Environment and Psychosomatic Diseases*. London, Oxford University Press, 1971, pp. 299-311.

61. Simon, A., Herbert, C.C., and Straus, R. (Eds.): *The Physiology of Emotions*. Springfield, Ill., Thomas, 1961.
62. Simon, H.A., and Newell, A.: The uses and limitations of models. In Marx, M.H. (Ed.): *Theories in Contemporary Psychology*. New York, Macmillan Co., 1964, p. 89.
63. Soderberg, U.: Short term reactions in the thyroid gland, revealed by continuous measurement of blood flow, rate of uptake of radioactive iodines and rate of release of labelled hormones. *Acta Physiol Scand*, 42 (147):5, 1958.
64. Tanner, J.M. (Ed.): *Stress and Psychiatric Disorder*. Oxford, Blackwell, 1960.
65. Teitelbaum, H.: *Psychosomatic Neurology*. New York, Grune and Stratton, 1964.
66. Tingley, J.O., Morris, A.W., and Hill, S.R.: Studies of the diurnal variation and response to emotional stress of the thyroid gland. *Clin Res*, 6:134, 1958.
67. Wolf, S., and Goodell, H. (Eds.): *Harold G. Wolff's "Stress and Disease."* Springfield, Ill., Thomas, 1968.
68. Wolff, H.G.: Stressors as a cause of disease in man. In Tanner, J.M. (Ed.): *Stress and Psychiatric Disorder*. Oxford, Blackwell, 1960, pp. 17-30.
69. ————: *Stress and Disease*. Springfield, Ill., Thomas, 1953.
70. Yates, F.E., and Maran, J.W.: Stimulation and inhibition of adrenocorticotropin (ACTH) release. In Sawyer, W., and Knobile, E. (Eds.): *Handbook of Physiology*. Section on Endocrinology, Hypothalamo-hypophyseal System. Am Physiol Soc, in press.

COMMENT

W. T. SINGLETON*

I would like to begin by paying tribute to Dr. Levi and his colleagues at the Karolinska Institute in Stockholm. Over the past decade they have given us a fine demonstration of research which cuts across academic boundaries between clinical medicine, biochemistry and behavior studies. Each of these areas has separate traditions and expertise. There are enormous problems in doing interdisciplinary research of this kind, partly to do with the sheer range of knowledge required and partly to do with the translation or matching problems across the boundaries. Dr. Levi and his colleagues have demonstrated that these problems can be overcome.

As a person interested in attempts to conceptualize human behavior I have been cautiously in favor of the concept of stress for a number of reasons.

1. At the philosophical level it incorporates or assumes two of the most fundamental ideas which we have been able to develop about human behavior: namely the concept of purpose and the concept of awareness. As Morgenstern[4] has pointed out, the basic difference between the natural sciences and the social sciences is that the latter do not make sense without the incorporation of the idea of purpose. On the question of awareness it has emerged that the basic differences between lower and higher forms of life are in the degree of awareness or consciousness and self-consciousness.

2. At the methodological level we need such ideas to rescue psychology from the worst rigors of the human experimental psychologists who have begun to think of human behavior almost as analogous to computer behavior—pure information processing with inputs, computation and outputs. We need to be reminded that apart from measures of performance as reflections of activity in the higher levels of

*Professor, University of Aston in Birmingham, United Kingdom.

the central nervous system, there are relevant measures of behavior in autonomic, endocrinal and muscular terms. In more colloquial terminology what a man is doing makes more sense when it is considered in the context of what he is trying to do, how important it is to him and how he feels about how well he is doing.

3. At the technique level the increasing utilization of measures of the internal state of the body have re-emphasized the importance of the essentially rhythmical nature of biological processes from the long cycles of lifetimes through to the circadian cycles. Measures of stress activity make more sense if they are seen as temporary shifts following the exigencies of the current situation superimposed on these basic rhythms.

In spite of these important dividends I am still only cautiously in favor of the concept of stress because it seems to me that it might well turn out to be a misconception rather than a conception, a digression rather than a progression in the advancement of knowledge of behavior for the following reasons.

1. I have elsewhere developed the point[6] that there is a disturbing similarity between concepts such as stress and arousal and older concepts such as fatigue and effort. With the advantages of hindsight it is now clear that these latter were abandoned after a few decades of research work because there were too many different ideas about their meaning and in consequence too many inconsistencies in research findings. Yet stress and arousal are no more precisely defined than were fatigue and effort.

As another example of the importance of defining terms we might consider the measurement of intelligence. The psychometricians have been aware of their inadequacies and inconsistencies in trying to define what they were trying to measure, but they honestly thought that if they pursued the measuring for long enough the definition would emerge. Of course it did not and it has not. The problem of intelligence has gotten more and more complicated and the measurement has gotten correspondingly more diffuse.[1] We are still nowhere near defining what we mean by the term in any sense which is reliable and valid. In practical terms, in Britain, the proposition that it is possible to measure or predict the qualities of young people by mental testing has created immeasurable misery, injustice and inefficiency within the educational system over the past thirty years. For behavioral variables at least the precision of definition predetermines the accuracy at measurement, and to pursue measurement in the hope of clarifying definition is a *fata morgana*. Furthermore we are not entitled to comment on broad aspects of ways of life unless we have developed a solid foundation of precise definitions and erected on it an impeccable structure of evidence. As private citizens we may make whatever contribution we think appropriate about the importance of stress levels in our civilization, but as scientists and technologists it would be irresponsible and perhaps mischievous to comment unless we can speak from the security of such a framework.

2. We also need to recognize that the natural scientists have developed a coherent respectable model of the physical world, and yet concepts from their field do not fit at all well with the concept of stress. Every valid stress measure depends on a clumsy weighted combination of physical measures. This is true even in the case of relatively simple environmental stressors. Heat stress for example depends on the ambient temperature, radiant temperature, humidity and wind speed. The available physical measures of noise are connected in what can only be described as a most devious fashion with the effects of noise on people. Perhaps there need be no necessary relationship between physical measurement and behavior measurement but one would feel more confident in biosocial concepts which matched more readily with our concepts of the physical world than does stress.

3. The relationship between biological and behavioral indices is equally complex. It already seems to be clear that there can be no single physiological or biological measure which can be regarded as an unambiguous index of stress in the psychological sense. In fact the relationship is sufficiently remote to warrant questioning whether there is any utility in trying to unify the psychological and biological meanings of stress. Psychologists have recently tried to clarify the field by distinguishing between stress and strain in a way analogous to that in which engineers use these terms, that is stress is the imposed situation and strain is the individual reaction to the situation. This, of course, is completely at variance with the biological concept of stress which has in recent years been dependent on the general adaptation syndrome.[7] In psychological terms this is not stress at all but strain.

4. Accepting that biological indications of stress are parameter

shifts superimposed on inherent periodic variations, the psychologist would feel happier if the biological attempts to measure these variables took more account of the periodic variations, for example by utilizing the mathematics of periodic and stochastic processes.

Inevitably, laboratory experiments concerning human reactions involve only a fragmentary measurement of the total activity and consequently they encourage a gross oversimplification of the origins of that activity. From the biological standpoint, as Dr. Levi has pointed out, the response to stress with its inherent preparation for flight or fight can best be explained in terms of the history of phylogenetic development. It was more adaptive to earlier modes of human behavior than it is today. From the cybernetic point of view[2] the organism can be conceived as a goal-seeking device and the current situation is interpreted in relation to goals. The individual is operating in a particular functional space, he will behave according to a purpose which will probably involve moving conditionally towards some end, conditionally in that not only are there goals he is pursuing but there are also negative goals he is avoiding. Added to this is the further complication that he has a hierarchy of needs[3] along which he may advance or regress depending on the stresses of the time. Thus stress can be seen as degree of interference with the pursuit of ends. In contrast, from the experimental psychologists' point of view[5] stress is effects on performance, e.g. effect on motion sickness, weightlessness, vibration, heat, noise, etc., or sometimes the effects of performance, e.g. vigilance, simultaneous tasks, speed, etc.

From the social psychologists' point of view[8] the experiment is a social situation within which both the subjects and the experimenters have interacting parts to play and stress is presumably a function of this interaction as well as other factors. The psychopathologist adds an additional complication in that the reaction to the situation may not be adaptive, the individual may remain healthy or may become schizoid or depressive (see later papers) depending on factors about which we have little understanding. We can of course agree that there are enormous individual differences. Admittedly these concepts are neither additive nor exclusive; we may eventually need all of them, none of them or parts of some of them. The point I am trying to make is that the current state of knowledge reveals some of the complexities of the problem but there has not yet been generated a universal model within which we can conceive the total problem.

In spite of these uncertainties we must obviously continue to do what we can, but in the current state of the art I believe that there is a real danger in over-generalization. We might do better to continue for some time to pursue isolated problems. We have a large variety of problems from preventive medicine to performance optimization and it is premature to try too hard to force all of these into a general theoretical framework which would inevitably be inadequate and would probably also be misleading.

Given that a general theory is not feasible at this stage it is even more unrealistic to attempt to prescribe remedies on the basis of theory. Taking Dr. Levi's model which involves the sequence: stressors/intervening variables/mechanisms/precursors of disease/disease, this model is entirely general and could for example have been applied to the study of dangers in cigarette smoking. It was possible to demonstrate correlations between frequency of exposure and relative incidence of various consequences, in other words correlations between smoking and the related diseases. The cause of the relationship in terms of mechanisms has still not been worked out, and it would have been impractical to wait for this knowledge to emerge before making recommendations about the dangers of cigarette smoking. The effects of stress are more complicated than the effects of cigarettes, and if this analogy is reasonable then it would seem optimal to proceed, for the moment, by putting most of our effort into looking for correlations rather than looking for mechanisms.

It must also be recognized that, in generating proposed remedies, we are relying on some assumptions about desirable ways and lengths of life which will not be universally agreed. I am reminded of a poem by Edna St. Vincent Millay:

> "My candle burns at both ends;
> It will not last the night;
> But ah, my foes, and oh my friends—
> It gives a lovely light."

While recognizing that these problems exist I hope that the conference will not digress too far into arguments about desirable ways of life since a sure way of stultifying a scientific conference is to spend too much time on what are essentially ethical and political problems.

Finally, and in summary, I would like to make some positive suggestions about how I think this field should be developed.

1. Let us for the moment solve a series of problems and get back to the theory when we have enough successful *ad hoc* solutions from which we can generalize.

2. The complexity of the variables involved is such that we are on safer ground in studying the real problems as they exist in the field rather than attempting to simulate them in a laboratory.

3. We should look for broad relationships or correlations on a macro scale rather than for causes or mechanisms on a micro scale.

4. We need longitudinal as well as lateral studies. The problems are not going to be solved completely within the next thirty years and we, therefore, have time to initiate projects from which we can expect to obtain useful new knowledge along this time scale.

5. Previous work has concentrated reasonably enough on extreme stress. There is also a great deal to be learned by looking at mild stress effects, particularly for combinations of stressors; for example the children in the hot noisy classroom or the businessmen in the noisy vibrating transport vehicle.

6. We need to look for adequate financial measures which are the ones most readily communicated to policy makers. The problem may be mainly to do with health and well-being but it is also to do with productivity, and here the important decision makers will listen more readily.

7. We need to study real problems which presently exist and to arrange our priorities in terms of their relative importance. It is too easy to merely study problems in terms of their relative ease of measurement. Remedies looking for diseases is not good technology.

REFERENCES

1. Butcher, H.J.: *Human Intelligence: Its Nature and Assessment.* London, Methuen, 1968.
2. McKay, D.M.: *Information, Mechanisms and Meaning.* Cambridge, Mass., MIT Press, 1969.
3. Maslow, A.H.: A theory of human motivation. *Psychol Rev, 50:*370-396, 1943.
4. Morgenstern, O.: Game theory: A new paradigm of social science. In Zwicky, F., and Wilson, A.G. (Eds.): *New Methods of Thought and Procedure.* Berlin, Springer-Verlag, 1967.
5. Poulton, E.C.: *Environment and Human Efficiency.* Springfield, Ill., Thomas, 1970.

Life Stress and Illness

6. Singleton, W.T.: The measurement of man at work with particular reference to arousal. In Singleton, W.T., Fox, J.G., and Whitfield, D. (Eds.): *Measurement of Man at Work.* London, Taylor and Francis, 1971.

7. Selye, H.: *The Stress of Life.* New York, McGraw-Hill, 1956.

8. Smith, P.B. (Ed.): *Group Processes.* Harmondsworth, Penguin, 1970.

Chapter III

PSYCHOSOCIAL FACTORS IN DISEASE: HYPOTHESES AND FUTURE RESEARCH

AUBREY KAGAN

L EVI HAS DEMONSTRATED in the previous chapter, by reference to work from his laboratory and to that of others, support for parts of the general concept that social factors may give rise to disease through the medium of higher nervous processes. I will try to look at future studies in the light of what he has said. My aim is towards prevention of ill health in man. I will bear in mind three of Professor Singleton's recommendations in his comments on Levi's presentation: solve real problems, get into the field and start large-scale prospective studies.

THE PRESENT SITUATION

For the last fifty years frequency, intensity and rapidity of spread of change in social relationships has been greater than ever before.[4] This tendency is likely to continue. Some of these changes are undoubtedly useful, but we suspect there are dangers. Our suspicion is particularly aroused because some of the social functions that are fundamental to individual and social life, and probably those most controlled by innate forces are affected, e.g. (1) the tendency to increase the distance between the decision makers and those affected by the decisions (large community, no personal knowledge of the leader, one-way communication from leader to led); (2) the tendency for individual status to be in doubt; (3) the tendency to require community loyalties at an international or multinational level when little loyalty is perceived beyond the subnational or national

41

level; (4) the tendency for the community not to perceive its loyalties to the individual; and (5) the changes in social attitudes toward pair bonding, sexual intercourse, reproduction, childrearing, male/female roles at home and at work, and overt male dominance.[6]

We are all aware of the spate of ill health, as well as the advantages, that came in the wake of social change during the Industrial Revolution. Our method of dealing with the dangers was, and still is, to recognize them usually after a large measure of damage has been done and to apply rational corrections. This method—sometimes called "planning from crisis to crisis"—is likely to be too slow and dangerous for the rate of change that exists today.

Our problem then is to understand the ways in which social change is beneficial or harmful and to plan rational action in advance in order to optimize the former and minimize the latter.

In the light of Levi's review, we may restate our general concept: social change gives rise to psychological stimuli which, under some circumstances (of psychobiological program and interacting variables), cause "Selye stress"* which, whether the emotional response be pleasant or unpleasant, will, under some circumstances (duration, frequency, intensity of Selye stress or type of physiological response to Selye stress or other interacting variables) will lead to precursors of disease or disease.

The evidence he brings forward for man demonstrates that social situations (Fig. II-1, Box 1) of certain types, acting for up to a few days, cause Selye stress (Fig. II-1, Boxes 1 and 3) and that this varies with the psychobiological program (Fig. II-1, Box 2). There is strong associative evidence (and in some cases proof) relating Selye stress to some precursors of disease (Fig. II-1, Boxes 4 and 5). The evidence that long-duration (several months) social change is associated with Selye stress (Fig. II-1, Boxes 1 and 3) is somewhat tenuous.

FUTURE DIRECTIONS

Thus, it is clear that the problem of "the role of social change in disease causation and prevention" is in a strategic area for research.[7] While there are many hypotheses, few have been adequately tested in men. There are insufficient data to show whether actions, such as those proposed twenty or thirty years ago by Spitz or Bowlby, are

*The term "Selye stress" is used throughout in the sense defined by Levi in Chapter II.

sufficiently effective, or free from danger, or that their cost in relation to benefit merits wide-spread application.

The goal of rational health action will be best served by testing hypotheses and evaluating health action. Three general types of hypotheses are proposed as ripe for testing: (1) control of psychosocial environment reduces disease; (2) control of psychological and/or physiological reactions reduces disease, and (3) these responses are interrelated and mediated through neuroendocrine mechanisms as a common pathway.

Within each of these general areas, we could specify a host of hypotheses. But the aim is to select those which are likely to be practicable and to give the greatest understanding of the problem.

The part of the system depicted in Figure II-1 which, if understood, would be most likely to lead to an understanding of the whole, is the mechanism. If the mechanisms were known and we could measure them we would have tools which could be used to: (1) judge whether a social situation, psychological stimulus or interacting factor was likely to be harmful or beneficial, and, thereby, we could reduce the number that need to be tested; (2) estimate which subjects were at high risk, thereby increasing the sensitivity of test situations and perhaps increasing efficiency of health action, and (3) make evaluation of health action less difficult.

Specific hypotheses concerning mechanisms that might be considered ready for testing in the light of Levi's review are: (1) Selye stress is a common pathway by which psychsocial stimuli cause disease; (2) to cause disease, Selye stress must be prolonged, frequent, intense or some combination of these; (3) disease does not follow Selye stress if the normal physiological responses for which it prepares the organism occur (activities connected with fight or flight), and (4) Selye stress is an index of response to stimulus but is not a disease mechanism.

To support such studies, development of methods for assessing Selye stress under habitual conditions, and for long periods, would be advantageous. These could include: (1) trying to establish whether response to a specific stimulus under laboratory conditions reflects response to stimuli of many different kinds under habitual conditions, and (2) establishing whether factors which can be assessed by socially acceptable monitoring instruments for periods of a day or up to a week can be used as an index of Selye stress. Some of this may have been established already.

Examples of hypotheses of social change, psychological stimuli and interacting factors that seem to me to be ripe for test are: (1) life change causes disease if, and only if, it gives rise to some aspect of* Selye stress; (2) life change which gives rise to psychological stimuli and some aspect of Selye stress does not give rise to disease if the psychological response is pleasant (e.g. achievement of something desired); (3) interacting factors which reduce some aspect of Selye stress reduce risk of disease, and (4) interacting factors which do not reduce or increase some aspect of Selye stress do not reduce or increase risk of disease.

SOME PROBLEMS IN TESTING HYPOTHESES AND EVALUATING HEALTH ACTIONS

Testing a hypothesis implies showing under what circumstances, if any, it is correct, and under what circumstances it is wrong. Evaluation of a health action embodies similar approaches, i.e. to show under what circumstances the action is effective, under what circumstances it is dangerous, and additionally some estimate of required cost.

The problems are ethical and technical.[5]

Ethics

The essential ethical problem is that evaluation is a form of experimentation. We do something, we are not quite sure what its effect will be, and we want to find out what happens. There is no doubt that this is an experiment, and there is equally no doubt, in my mind, that unbridled experimentation might be and has been both dangerous and harmful to the subject. However, it is not necessary to treat people like guinea pigs in order to carry out experiments. Under certain conditions, experimentation is both reasonable and ethical. The conditions are that the subject should know what the experiment is about, what can be done and the reasons why, and then should be free to volunteer or refrain. The experiment must be carried out in a humane way and everything must be done to minimize dangers to a level that the ordinary person is accustomed to take during his ordi-

*The words "some aspects of" are used as a short form of reference to intensity, frequency, duration or some combination of these, or Selye stress not followed by flight/fight type of activities.

nary life activities. Not only should all this be done, but, to use the words of Hailsham (in a sense that he did not intend) "should be seen to be done." Preferably, the problem should be of importance to the people taking part in the experiment. Under these circumstances, experimentation is ethical and we should not hesitate to say so, nor should we disguise our intention to experiment by using words such as "intervention" or "controlled trial." The obverse of the situation is that all action that is unevaluated is an experiment, but carried out in such a way that we cannot learn from the experiment. In my opinion, that is unethical.

Technical Problems

Technically, the present situation is due to inherent difficulties in the problems to be tackled that are unlikely to be met without modification of traditional methods.

The usual process of discovery depends upon thought, observation and experiment. Thought directs observation along a particular pathway. Observation sends thoughts in a particular direction. These processes lead to a hypothesis which is then tested. The results of this lead to an acceptable theory or one that needs further test, or a change in hypothesis, or a set of observations is indicated, and so on.

There is an element of chance in choosing the right observation, the right hypothesis, the right conditions for observation and the right test situation. That is why the majority of ideas and hypotheses prove to be sterile, and chance observations may be productive.

A negative result is only useful if the false hypothesis is in some way related to the correct hypothesis and its disproof directs attention to the latter, or, if by excluding one of a few possibilities, attention is directed to the others In any event, unless the first hypothesis is luckily correct, observation and experimentation have to be repeated.

This process has succeeded and is tolerable when the procession between thought, observation, experiment and back again is fast and inexpensive. A train of thought can be followed, modified, retested or cast aside, and a new idea can then be put through the same process. Under these conditions the process results in discovery sufficiently often to receive acclaim and acceptance and to have resulted in the undoubted advances of science that we now experience.

When the process is slowed down, e.g. smaller chances of getting the right idea, or need for large-scale prolonged observation and tests, the frequency of getting useful results is greatly diminished. The expense of procession becomes great and the expense of repetition enormous in terms of manpower, materials and time.

The latter situation describes our predicament. Here the number of factors suspected, and, therefore, to be observed, is great. Observation of representative samples of large numbers of human beings under habitual conditions is required. The number of possible associations is great because not only are the number of suspected factors large but it is likely that combinations of factors should be examined. The number of hypotheses arising is large. Tests of hypotheses of prevention of disease seldom take less than two years and often take longer. Discovery is the exception. False hypotheses leading to sterile results are the rule. Repetition of the process becomes necessary but inexpedient in terms of effort, time and money.

We cannot do without the iterative process of "thought, observation, test." We must make it more effective. This might be achieved by: (1) improving study designs; (2) better forms of mathematical analysis of data; (3) greater, and known, precision of observation; (4) more efficient assessment of larger numbers of subjects, and (5) multipurpose action, i.e. several hypotheses or health actions tested simultaneously and many observations made at the same time which, by suitable analysis, will enlarge our understanding of the whole system.

In particular, attention should be paid to: (1) the definition of relevant factors; (2) the definition and testing and modification of methods for assessing these factors and establishing their precision and bias; (3) the problem of control groups; (4) the achievement of high response and adherence to the study; (5) follow-up; (6) numbers of subjects and (7) costs.

I will not deal with the first here except to say that, usually, factors connected with safety and cost and ways in which the action is dangerous are forgotten.

Methods for measuring various factors and the ways in which these can be improved and tested for precision and bias have, in recent years, been fairly well established. At any rate, the principles are now available for doing this. So are the principles for reducing bias when it cannot be tolerated. One point can be emphasized here.

It is now popular to refer to "the process of standardization," by which is meant carrying out measurements in a uniform way with the same kinds of instruments. This is sometimes useful but does not necessarily lead to precision or lack of bias. The essential feature is "calibration." For this, standards are necessary and when these are available or made available, then any kind of instrument in any person's hand may be calibrated so that it is comparable with any other kind of instrument in any other person's hand. One other point that needs mentioning is that it is not sufficient simply to establish procedures for measuring relevant factors. It is necessary during the course of a study to exert continuous "quality control." Principles for all this have now been set out.

The kinds of controls that have been used are: randomization of individuals to the "treated" or the "control" groups, historical controls and natural situations. Of these, the first, apart from exceptional circumstances, is the most reliable method. It is, however, rather difficult to arrange. Some notable examples in which this has been achieved in testing the effect of treatment on subjects and the effect of mass health screening, can be mentioned. One approach, which, perhaps, could be described as the "heroic" is where doctors are persuaded that random assignment of patients to "case" and "control" is reasonable. For example, this has been done in the treatment of the acute coronary case—whether "out-patient" injection of varicose veins is as good as or better than "in-patient" surgery[10]—and is being used at the moment to evaluate the effect of clofibrate on subjects with raised serum cholesterol in primary prevention of coronary heart disease.[10] A less heroic but very ingenious way is being used in the evaluation of mass health screening. In London, England,[2] and Titograd, Yugoslavia,[1] random samples of individuals of a particular community have been assigned to a regime of mass health screening and the controls to a regime of the traditional medical approach. These two groups will be compared for mortality, morbidity, disability, utilization of health services and costs of health services. This clever procedure has also been used in New York, USA,[9] to establish the value of mass health screening for cancer of the breast. Here, it is obviously unethical to screen a large group of women and assign at random those in whom cancer has been found to treatment and nontreatment groups. It is quite ethical, however, to invite a random half of a large group of women to take part in a screening program and to compare the kinds of cases that are found by the screening procedure and the usual procedures as well as the ultimate effect on the individual. There are notable difficulties in this procedure, but it appears that they can be overcome.

Problems of response are now fairly well known, and it seems that if one approaches almost any community in a manner that is in keeping with, and not against, their cultural mores and traditions, and if one treats them as human beings, something of the order of 80 percent will respond. Of the remaining 20 percent, if one takes care to make individual enquiries into the reasons for nonresponse, it is usually possible to reduce it to 10 percent without much difficulty. After this, improvement of the response rate becomes difficult and may not be worth the effort. Little is known about adherence, especially to unpleasant, uncomfortable or prolonged regimes.

How are people motivated to take part in an experiment? I think that there is a large body of data that might give us insight into this, particularly in efforts to study the effects of reduction of cigarette smoking and the taking of drugs to prevent high blood cholesterol, glucose intolerance, or high blood pressure, but this needs to be analyzed.

The problem of follow-up and numbers of subjects and costs are all related. If a study is to continue for three or four years, it is rather important to carry it out on a population that is not going to move very much during that time. Many populations do not come into this category but quite a number do. It is necessary to investigate this point before a study starts, and it is necessary to incorporate into the study design some arrangement for keeping in contact with the subjects even if they do move. Evaluation of health action often requires a very large number of man-years of study—something of the order of 50,000 to 100,000. There are several ways in which this number can be efficiently reduced. These are by improved precision, by characterizing each subject for each factor studied, by studies of high risk subjects, and by better choice of endpoints. It may also be assisted by developments in application of mathematics to the analysis of the data.

A little more could be said here on the subjects of "high risk" and choice of "endpoints." It is very clear that if the incidence of the endpoint (disease) in the "treated" and the "controls" is 1 percent and ½ percent per annum respectively, then a very large number of man-years of study will be required. If this could be increased to 15 percent and 7 percent, the number of man-years could be reduced considerably. This can be done sometimes by choosing high risk subjects. Of course, there is a price to pay which is that the study does not cover all kinds of persons at risk to the disease.

Another approach is by choosing an endpoint which is likely to have a very high incidence in the "treated" and a very low incidence in the "controls" or vice versa. This may require using one endpoint as the key indicator and two or three other supporting endpoints. An example could be given for the evaluation of prevention of coronary heart disease by reduction of high blood pressure or high blood cholesterol. It would be possible to conceive a study in which the treated and untreated were compared for incidence of coronary heart disease, incidence of all disease, mortality from all disease. The difference would be of the order of 3 or 4 or 5 percent, compared with 1, 2 or 3 percent. This would be difficult to show. But, supposing a third endpoint were included, namely, the frequency and extent of myocardial infarction in subjects who died in the treated and untreated: the differences are likely to be of the order of 10 percent and 80 percent, and this could be shown in relatively few cases. Of course, it could only be shown in the deaths, and there would be relatively few deaths. But calculations have shown that, if one were concerned with middle-aged males aged 50 ± 5 years, and the treatment reduced the incidence and mortality of coronary heart disease by 50 percent, then it is very likely that with as few as 6,000 man-years of study it would be shown that the treated had less myocardial infarction than the untreated. With the same amount of material, it would be possible to say that the incidence and mortality of coronary heart disease and other disease was no greater in the treated than the untreated, and the conclusion that the treatment was effective in reducing myocardial infarction could be drawn. This sort of reasoning is somewhat speculative, but is based on information from population-related autopsy data and is quite likely to be correct. If so, a study could be reduced from the generally accepted level of 100,000 man-years to something of the order of 6,000 or, to be on the safe side, 10,000 man-years—a 90 percent saving.

Analysis is greatly strengthened by precise data and adequate controls. When sufficient data are available to show interrelationships between the parts of the system, it may be possible to use systems analysis techniques to simulate the whole system and show how it works under different conditions.

One of the many reasons given for the failure to evaluate health actions is the high cost. Can this be reduced? Is it really high? One of the striking features of many health actions that need to be evaluated is that many of the expensive features for different problems overlap. For example, it would be possible to choose a dozen problems that could be carried out in the same sample frame, in the same sample of subjects, by the same observers and in the same places. Many of the observations would be in common, but a few additional ones peculiar to each problem would have to be added. The number of subjects would have to be increased but the facilities for followup would be the same. I have made calculations elsewhere[3] which indicate that a dozen problems tackled separately might cost something in the region of $20,000,000, while tackled together they would cost only $8,000,000. Multipurpose testing is extremely likely to reduce the cost. Furthermore, by including additional observations related to the problems under study, useful information may be obtained for very little additional cost. But is the cost of evaluation really high? The cost of not evaluating can be enormous in actual money spent, in money wasted and, above all, in harm done. Since nearly all our health measures are expensive and dangerous, we can assume that money spent on evaluation will be repaid. It is a little like our policy with regard to buying a house or anything else that is rather expensive. Before buying it, we get an expert to decide what its weaknesses and merits are. We are prepared to spend perhaps 1 percent of the total cost on this, and that would be a very reasonable expenditure for evaluation of health actions. One factor that has changed appreciably the cost and feasibility of multipurpose health actions is the development of technology for examining large numbers of people for large numbers of factors. To my mind, this evaluation is the proper use for automated multiphasic health testing at the present time.

FUTURE RESEARCH
Strategy

A number of participants have indicated limitations of retrospective studies, some of which can be overcome by prospective studies. Both methods can only suggest hypotheses or give support or the contrary for existing hypotheses. Prospective studies give clearer results and better information on the interrelation of numerous factors than retrospective studies, but are more expensive.

However, by including experimental approaches in a prospective study, hypotheses may be tested and health actions evaluated. This implies altering some of the conditions in Boxes 1, 3, 4 or 6 of Figure II-1 in a subgroup of subjects, and not altering them in another subgroup which is used as a control. Comparison of events in the "altered" and "control" subgroups tests the effect of the alteration. This, given suitable conditions, is only a little more difficult than observational/analytical prospective studies, but the ethical and technical conditions mentioned in the previous section must be observed.

A number of health workers, inspired by reports from business and industry, believe that "systems analysis" will give a deep and broad understanding of health problems in a shorter period of time. This certainly remains to be demonstrated for health problems (and for all but a few types of industrial problems). However, if one could develop a mathematical model of the whole system (see Fig. II-1) that could be used to simulate the real situation, it would be a useful way of understanding what would happen to the various parts of the system under very many different conditions. This possibility is worth exploring.

In my view, the best way of attempting this is to obtain a good idea of the interrelationships of the parts of the system (Fig. II-1) by experiment and observation, to translate these into mathematical terms, and to relate forecasts derived from simulation to observations of real events. The observations for this can be included with little extra expenditure into a prospective experimental study.

The strategy advocated, therefore, is a prospective experimental study in which several hypotheses concerning mechanism, stimulus or interacting variables, are tested, and, at the same time, observations are made of the interrelationships of many other factors included in the boxes in Figure II-1.

Example

Here I will give a rough outline of two studies of the type described above that are likely to be ethical, possible and useful, and, at the same time, test some elements of the general concept that control of psychosocial stimuli and their effects prevents ill health.

Day-care Nurseries and the Health of Children

This question is of growing importance in those communities where husband and wife are encouraged to work away from home. Many countries have set up day-care facilities for young children, but little is known of the advantages or disadvantages of different forms of day-care for the health of the child and its family. No one knows whether different children require different forms of day-care.

Hypotheses to be tested: (1) Large classes are not harmful for any child; (2) large classes are not harmful for children without siblings; (3) large classes are not harmful for children who are low adrenalin secretors, and (4) additional physical exercise or teacher guidance protects the health of children who are high adrenalin secretors if adrenalin secretion is thereby reduced.

We will seek to see if there are optimum levels of adrenalin secretion for health; interrelationships between factors will be determined, and association between change in health and attitudes of the child and change in health and attitudes of the parents and siblings will be sought.

Social Situation. Day-care nurseries will be of two types: large classes of twenty children and small classes of four children. Each nursery should have at least two classes. With two classes per nursery we will need about ten large class nurseries and thirty small class nurseries.

Psychobiological Program. Children will be divided into high and low adrenalin secretors by response to a standard load-test.

Mechanism. Stress will be assessed at frequent intervals in terms of urinary epinephrine and 17-hydroxycorticosteroids. Other factors may be assessed.

Precursors. Changes in growth, nutritional status, attitudes and conflicts of child and siblings; attitudes and conflicts of parents and family economy.

DISEASE. Disability of child, siblings and parents. Specific diseases in child, siblings and parents.

INTERACTING VARIABLES. These will include siblings versus no siblings which will be presumed to act on the social situation to affect the stimulus; physical exercise added or teacher guidance added versus physical exercise reduced or teacher guidance not added which will be presumed to act on the mechanism to affect stress.

Other interacting variables that will be assessed are: family characteristics (number of parents, social class, type of dwelling); life change events in family; and personal characteristics (iq, attitudes, past and present health of parent, siblings and child).

The study design will be (a) to randomly assign children in need of day nursery care to large and small class schools; (b) each school child assigned to that school will be randomly assigned to each of the two classes, one of which will have physical exercise added or teacher guidance added and the other will have physical exercise reduced or teacher guidance not added; in small classes it will be necessary, and in large classes it may be necessary, to ensure stratification or equal proportions of children with siblings and children with no siblings and high adrenalin secretors and low adrenalin secretors; (c) adrenalin secretion and other interacting variables will be assessed for all children before assignment to the day nursery, and (d) precursors and disease should be assessed in children of similar social class, etc., who do not need day-care as well as in the test children and in their families.

Life-change Events and the Health of Young Adults

Here an attempt will be made to see if the association of minor life change events and minor disease, which has been demonstrated by Rahe et al.,[8] is causative and, if so, whether it depends on pleasantness or unpleasantness of the events, the strength of the psychological stimulus, the strength of the mechanism (or response) or on factors interacting with the response.

The importance of this type of study is its relevance to the general concept of the role of psychological stimuli arising from social situations in the onset of ill health. It seeks to differentiate between types of life change events. This is likely to be possible because the events and the illnesses are relatively minor.

The hypotheses to be tested will be: (1) when all life change events are reduced, disability is reduced; (2) this is independent of whether the life change events are pleasant, indifferent or unpleasant; (3) disability is associated with the difference between expectation and perceived situation; (4) disability is associated with Selye stress; (5) disability is always reduced by exercise response to Selye stress; (6) reduction of disability by exercise response to Selye stress depends on the level of all life change events; (7) reduction of disease disability by exercise response depends on change in level of Selye stress, and (8) reduction of disease disability by exercise response depends on the level of difference between expectation and perceived situation.

In addition, interrelationships will be determined for: (a) pleasant, indifferent, unpleasant and total life change events on the one hand with "difference between expectation and perceived situation" and Selye stress; (b) the difference between expectation and perceived situation with Selye stress and disability, and (c) other interacting variables with the difference between expectation and perceived situation, Selye stress, and disability.

SOCIAL SITUATION. Young men under close observation for a period of a few months, e.g. sailors at sea, will be artificially exposed to extra life change events of a pleasant, unpleasant or indifferent nature. For others, life change events will be reduced. A psychological stimulus representing the difference between what each person expects and each thinks his situation to be will be assessed.

PSYCHOBIOLOGICAL PROGRAM. Each person taking part in the study will be tested for: (a) events he finds pleasant, unpleasant or indifferent; (b) adrenalin response to a standard load test; (c) ability to habituate and (d) temperament.

MECHANISMS. Selye stress will be assessed at frequent intervals. Other related factors may also be assessed.

PRECURSORS. Heart rate, blood pressure, leukocyte count, erythrocyte count, sedimentation rate, serum cholesterol, glucose tolerance, attitudes and conflicts will be assessed at frequent intervals.

DISABILITY. All specific disease, disability and attendance for medical advice will be recorded.

INTERACTING VARIABLES. A method of applying substitute "fight/flight" activity will be devised (exercise response). Other interacting variables, such as age, type of work, exposure to heat, noise, etc., will be determined.

Study Design

After an initial period of one month's exposure to a low level of life change, men will be randomly assigned pleasant, indifferent, unpleasant or reduced life change events subgroups. It may be necessary to stratify for each type of work, etc.

Those in the pleasant events subgroup will be exposed for a period of time to an excess of pleasant situations (the situations will be tailored to what is known about each man). Those in indifferent and unpleasant subgroups will be similarly exposed to an excess of indifferent and unpleasant situations, respectively. Those assigned to reduced life change subgroups will be protected from exposure to life change events.

In each type of subgroup, men will be assigned at random to two groups. One will receive exercise, the other will receive a placebo. The difference between expectation and perceived situation, Selye stress, pleasant events and disease disability will be assessed at frequent intervals.

It may be possible to repeat the experiment with change of assignment to subgroup, e.g. from pleasant to unpleasant, from unpleasant to pleasant, from indifferent to reduced life changes, etc.

CONCLUSIONS

The foregoing discussion points out the urgency and importance of an understanding of the ways in which psychological stimuli arising from social change can cause or prevent disease. A model of the system and interaction of the parts of the system were described earlier by Levi (Fig. II-1), and the elements were defined.

It is pointed out, and this is confirmed by other investigators, that notions of association between social events and disease have been supported quite strongly by studies of a wide range of life events in young men with subsequent minor disease, in older men recovered from myocardial infarction with subsequent death, in women with subsequent nonendogenous depression, and in high risk subjects with schizophrenic episodes.

Several investigators have shown that subjective ratings of life events vary considerably between individuals and possibly within individuals at different periods of time. It is therefore necessary to devise better ways of quantifying life change events in individuals and of assessing the stimulus in the individual.

I mention the psychological stimuli of threat and ambiguity and focus on the difference between expectation and the perceived situation. Other participants will emphasize the likely importance of these stimuli.

I indicate the need to move from studies of association to studies of hypotheses testing. The guidelines for ethical approaches to this task, and the technical requirements and reasons for choosing multi-hypotheses-testing prospective studies with additional observations that may make it possible to construct a mathematical model of the system, are set forth.

The key hypotheses concern mechanisms and important hypotheses relate to causative stimuli (and the social situations that produce them) and protective interacting factors.

Two examples of studies that might test such hypotheses within the general strategy of prospective experimental studies in which observations are simultaneously made on parts of interrelations of the "system" are given in rough outline.

Data published by some of the participants of this Symposium support the possibility of such studies, e.g. the short interval between life change events (one month) and minor illness in young men; attacks of schizophrenia in those at high risk; death in those recovered from myocardial infarction; the high incidence of deprivation and adaptive disorder in women; and the possibility of following a large number of middle-aged men, some of whom could be protected from or supported during life change events.

My conclusion is that if some of these threads can be picked up and studied along the lines suggested, much progress is likely to be made in understanding ways of handling social change so as to increase benefit and reduce harm.

REFERENCES

1. Djordjevic, D.: Personal communication, 1970.
2. Holland, W.W.: Personal communication, 1971.
3. Kagan, A.R.: Automated Multiphasic Health Testing (AMHT) in re-

search. World Health Organization Internal Document ENCD/70.3, 1970.

4. ————: Epidemiology and society, stress and disease. In Levi, L. (Ed.): *Society, Stress and Disease: The Psychosocial Environment and Psychosomatic Diseases*. London, Oxford University Press, 1971, pp. 36-48.

5. ————: Evaluation of mass screening for health: Needs, difficulties and possibilities. *J Public Health, 86*:119-124, 1972.

6. ————: *Society, Stress and Disease: The Productive and Reproductive Age—Male and Female Roles and Relationships*. In press.

7. ————, and Levi, L.: Health and environment: Psychosocial stimuli—a review. *Soc Sci Med*, in press.

8. Rahe, R.H., Gunderson, E.K.E., and Arthur, R.J.: Demographic and psychosocial factors in acute illness reporting. *J Chronic Dis, 23*:245-255, 1970.

9. Shapiro, S., Strax, P., and Venet, L.: Evaluation of periodic breast cancer screening with mamography. *JAMA, 196*:731-738, 1966.

10. Wilson, J.M.G., and Cochrane, A.C.: Personal communication, 1970.

Chapter IV

LIFE CHANGE AND SUBSEQUENT ILLNESS REPORTS

Richard H. Rahe

INTRODUCTION

MAN'S SUSCEPTIBILITY to illness is determined both by his constitutional endowment and by temporal factors in his life experience. Constitutional characteristics, both genetic and acquired, operate throughout an individual's lifetime. Constitutional endowment helps to explain an individual's susceptibilities to particular types of illnesses but does little to explain why an individual develops an illness at a particular point in time. Investigations into the timing of illness onset often, therefore, focus upon factors occurring in subjects' lives shortly prior to recognized illness. Recent exposure to a virulent strain of adenovirus is, for example, a temporal factor of importance in explaining why a subject has just developed a "cold."

Recent life changes are another example of temporal phenomena of apparent psychophysiologic importance in the precipitation of illnesses. Recent life changes appear to act as "stressors" partially accounting for illness onset.[10,13,16,21,22] Conversely, when subjects' lives are in a relatively steady state of psychosocial adjustment with few ongoing life changes, little or no illness tends to be reported.[10,13,22]

At the U.S. Navy Medical Neuropsychiatric Research Unit, San Diego, California, recent life changes data have been gathered on nearly four thousand subjects, and these and other data have been examined for their significance in the precipitation of illness. Individuals studied have included approximately 2,500 U.S. Navy enlisted men aboard three heavy cruisers, 50 Navy and Marine Corps personnel discharged with psychiatric disabilities, approximately 250 U.S. Navy Underwater Demolition Team (UDT) trainees, and slightly less than 1,000 Royal Norwegian Navy enlisted men. The review to follow concentrates on the utility of a life changes questionnaire for predicting near-future illness, although other predictors of illness are briefly mentioned in the Discussion.

METHODOLOGY
The Schedule of Recent Experience (SRE)
Life Changes Questionnaire

Researchers at the University of Washington in Seattle constructed the early editions of the Schedule of Recent Experience (SRE) questionnaire in order to systematically document clinically observed life events reported by subjects during the years prior to developing (respiratory) illnesses.[3] The design of the SRE has always been to include a broad spectrum of recent life changes, including personal, social, occupational and family areas of life adjustment.

For many years no allowances were made for the relative degrees of life change inherent in the various life events included in the SRE. One life change, such as death of a spouse, was given the same value as another life change, such as residential move. In 1964, a scaling experiment to reflect the various degrees of life change inherent in different SRE items was carried out.[10]

The forty-two life change questions contained in the SRE were scaled according to the proportionate scaling methods of Stevens.[27] A sample of nearly 400 subjects of both sexes and of differing ages, race, religion, education, social class, marital status and generation in the United States were selected. They were instructed that one of the life change events, marriage, had been arbitrarily assigned a life change unit (LCU) value of 500. The subjects then were instructed to assign LCU values for all of the remaining life change events in the SRE, using marriage as their reference. Other LCU values were to be proportionate to the 500 LCU arbitrarily assigned to marriage. For example, when a subject evaluated a life change event such as change in residence, he was to ask himself: "Is a change in residence more, less, or perhaps equal to the amount and duration of life change and readjustment inherent in marriage?" If he decided it was more, he was to indicate how much more by choosing a proportionately larger LCU value than the 500 assigned to marriage. If he decided it was less, he was to indicate how much less by choosing a proportionately smaller number than 500. If he decided it was equal, he was to assign 500 LCU. This process was repeated for each of the remaining life change events in the SRE questionnaire.[10]

Since this original scaling experiment, life changes scaling studies have been performed in other locations in the United States and in several other countries. Results from all of these life changes scaling experiments have been strikingly similar.[11] Most divergent results have been found between a small sample of Mexican-Americans and white, middle-class Americans and between a sample of Swedish subjects living in Stockholm and comparable Seattlites.[6,19] Table IV-I presents the list of the originally compiled forty-two life change events and their (Seattle) LCU values.

TABLE IV-I LIFE CHANGE EVENTS

		LCU Values
Family:	Death of spouse	100
	Divorce	73
	Marital separation	65
	Death of close family member	63
	Marriage	50
	Marital reconciliation	45
	Major change in health of family	44
	Pregnancy	40
	Addition of new family member	39
	Major change in arguments with wife	35
	Son or daughter leaving home	29
	In-law troubles	29
	Wife starting or ending work	26
	Major change in family get-togethers	15
Personal:	Detention in jail	63
	Major personal injury or illness	53
	Sexual difficulties	39
	Death of a close friend	37
	Outstanding personal achievement	28
	Start or end of formal schooling	26
	Major change in living conditions	25
	Major revision of personal habits	24
	Changing to a new school	20
	Change in residence	20
	Major change in recreation	19

	Major change in church activities	19
	Major change in social activities	18
	Major change in sleeping habits	16
	Major change in eating habits	15
	Vacation	13
	Christmas	12
	Minor violations of the law	11
Work:	Being fired from work	47
	Retirement from work	45
	Major business adjustment	39
	Changing to different line of work	36
	Major change in work responsibilities	29
	Trouble with boss	23
	Major change in working conditions	20
Financial:	Major change in financial state	38
	Mortgage or loan over $10,000	31
	Mortgage foreclosure	30
	Mortgage or loan less than $10,000	17

The practical result of these LCU weightings has been that recent life change events could be given quantitative values reflecting the average degree or intensity of life change. Arbitrary time intervals over which life changes (LCU) were summed in order to compute incidence rates included two years, one year, six months, three months, one week and one day in search of the most appropriate time interval for illness prediction.[5, 10, 13, 22, 23, 28]

RESULTS
RECENT LIFE CHANGES AND NEAR-FUTURE ILLNESSES—EARLY RETROSPECTIVE STUDIES

Pilot studies conducted by the author while at the University of Washington in Seattle (1962 to 1965) had been generally retrospective in nature. Subjects studied were requested to review their life changes and illness histories over the ten preceding years and record these data on the SRE. There appeared to be little falloff in completeness of recording due to difficulty in remembering events or illnesses occurring several years prior to the study compared to more recent years. In these retrospective studies, an increase in subjects' LCU values during the year or two prior to their reported illnesses was found.[10] A wide variety of illnesses was reported—infections, accidents, metabolic disease and even exacerbations of congenital maladies. The observed buildup in subjects' life change intensity (LCU) prior to reported health changes appeared to be nonspecific, that is, without regard to type of ensuing health change. There did appear to be a positive relationship between the LCU intensity recorded by subjects during the year or two prior to illness and the severity of the subsequent illness.[10,22]

It was from this pilot study that the first quantitative estimate of how many LCU a subject might experience and still remain healthy was made.[10] The majority of the physician subjects who recorded 150 LCU or less a year reported good health for the succeeding year. When subjects' yearly LCU values ranged between 150 and 300 LCU, it was noted that an illness was reported during the following year in approximately half the cases. Finally, for the relatively few subjects who registered more than 300 LCU per year, an illness was recorded during the following year in 70 percent of the cases. It was also noted that illnesses which followed subjects' yearly LCU values of more than 300 tended to be multiple. This tendency was not seen for illnesses following lesser yearly LCU totals. Therefore, not only was an association noted between the magnitude of subjects' yearly LCU totals and the likelihood of subsequent illness but also the likelihood of experiencing multiple illnesses.

Beginning in 1965, a large-scale Navy retrospective study of life changes and illness was performed utilizing nearly 2,500 U.S. Navy enlisted men comprising virtually the entire ship's companies of three cruisers. Subjects were given the SRE questionnaire and requested to report both their life changes and their illness experience over the previous four years. These four years were divided into eight six-month intervals. Subjects' LCU totals were based on six-month intervals rather than a year's time as was done in previous studies.[13] Whenever an illness was reported by a subject over the four years under study, the six-month interval in which it occurred was labeled the "illness period." Subjects' LCU totals for all illness periods were examined along with their LCU totals for the two six-month intervals immediately prior to the illness period and the two six-month intervals immediately following the illness period, *provided that subjects were in good health during these peri-illness intervals.* For comparative purposes, all subjects who were healthy over the entire four years under investigation provided a six-month grand mean LCU value which was considered the best estimate of a "healthy baseline" LCU value.

The mean six-month LCU total for the illness period was found to be 174. Six months prior to the illness period, the subsequently ill subjects reported a mean LCU total of 125. Six months prior to this, these subjects had a mean LCU total of 100. Therefore, a gradual buildup in subjects' six-month LCU totals was seen over the 1½ years leading to the onset of illness. The ill subjects' six-month LCU magnitudes for the two six-month intervals following their illness period were 120 and 130. It appeared, therefore, that ill subjects' six-month LCU totals remained elevated over the year following their illness. In comparison, the six-month LCU healthy baseline value derived for all subjects reportedly in good health over the four-year time span was 85.[13]

Perhaps the best retrospective study of life changes and subsequent illness in terms of eliminating researcher bias was a small study of fifty Navy and Marine Corps personnel discharged from service for psychiatric illness incurred while on active duty.[22] In this study the life changes data, as well as the men's health records, had been compiled five years earlier by social workers and physicians who knew nothing of our research. Each change of duty station, marriage, combat experience, childbirth, divorce, severe financial difficulty, etc., was recorded in the men's personnel records or elicited by interview at the time of psychiatric evaluation prior to establishing disability. The men's health records, at times, extended over thiry years. All life changes which we thought were symptomatic of an illness or the direct result of an illness were omitted from the analyses. Yearly LCU totals calculated for each subject during each year he was in the military were then compared with his illness experiences. Illnesses were scaled according to severity on a scale of 1 to 5 reflecting the risk of death or permanent disability after a method devised by Hinkle.[4] In this study of fifty Navy and Marine Corps subjects, we found that the mean LCU yearly total for the year prior to illnesses of minor severity was 130. The mean LCU total recorded for the year prior to health changes of major severity was 164. In comparison, the mean yearly LCU value for all years studied was just 72. A significant increase in yearly LCU total was, therefore, evidenced the year prior to subjects' recorded health changes. In addition, a positive relationship was seen between LCU magnitude the year prior to an illness and the severity of that illness. Two instances of high yearly LCU totals occurring prior to death were also seen.[22]

These early retrospective studies complemented one another. For all samples it appeared that around 150 LCU per year (specifically, 85 LCU per six-month period) was a value reported by people who generally remained healthy over the following year. When a subject reported an illness, his concomitant LCU total was often seen to be twice this healthy baseline value, that is, more than 300 LCU per year. LCU totals in the year prior to illness, as well as in the year following illness, were significantly elevated over the healthy baseline totals. It was also seen that the LCU buildup during the year prior to illness—generally between 150 to 300 LCU/year—was particularly noticeable during the final six-month interval. Thus, for purposes of illness prediction, subjects' most recent six-month LCU totals appeared to be the optimum values to use.

RECENT LIFE CHANGES AND NEAR-FUTURE ILLNESSES—EARLY AND RECENT PROSPECTIVE STUDIES

In the original pilot study, a small prospective experiment was built into the research design.[10] Eighty-four of the eighty-eight physician-subjects were contacted nine months after completion of the life changes questionnaire and queried about their health change experiences during the past nine-month interval. Forty-one of the eighty-four subjects had indicated at the time of their completion of the SRE questionnaire that they had experienced at least 250 LCU during the preceding year's time. Twenty-four of these forty-one subjects, or 59 percent reported a health change during the nine-month followup interval. Thirty-two subjects had indicated that for the year prior to the SRE examination they had accumulated between 150 and 250 LCU. Eight of this group of thirty-two subjects, or 25 percent, reported a subsequent health change over the nine-month followup interval. Of the eleven remaining subjects who reported less than 150 LCU for the year prior to completing the SRE questionnaire, only one reported a health change during the followup interval.

Navy Shipboard Studies

Large-scale prospective studies of recent life changes and near-future illnesses were conducted utilizing enlisted crew members of three U.S. Navy cruisers.[2,10,12,16,20,21] Aboard ship there is only one medical facility where all health records are kept. Thus, medical criterion data could be obtained from standardized medical records rather than subjects' reports as was the case in the resident physician study. In addition, naval ships form natural ecologic units, and the crews tend to be homogeneous in terms of age, education and social backgrounds. The men, as a group, encounter nearly identical environmental conditions, temporal stresses, food sources and water supplies.

The enlisted men aboard these three large cruisers provided recent life changes information for the six months prior to overseas deployment and were followed to determine recorded illnesses during the ensuing six-month cruise period. Gastrointestinal, genitourinary, musculoskeletal and dermal disorders accounted for 80 percent of all illnesses recorded aboard the three cruisers.[16,21] Virtually all of these illnesses were minor in severity. Hence, this prospective study ultimately determined whether or not life change information for six months prior to going to sea could predict minor illnesses recorded during an overseas cruise.

LCU scores for life changes during the six months prior to overseas deployment were grouped into deciles. Decile groups with similar illness rates were then combined resulting in a final grouping of the sample into four divisions roughly approximating quartiles. The illness rates for the four divisions were: 7.7 illnesses/1000 men/day for LCU deciles 1 to 3 (low scores), 8.5 illnesses/1000 men/day for deciles 4 and 5, 9.2 illnesses 1000/men/day for deciles 6 to 8, and 9.9 illnesses/1000 men/day for deciles 9 and 10. An analysis of variance of the differences in illness incidence among the four groups was significant at the 0.01 probability level.

A companion analysis of the same prospective data divided the sample according to specific LCU score intervals based on the year prior to the overseas cruise. In other words, men who reported less than 100 LCU for the year prior to the cruise were included in one group, men who recorded between 101 and 200 LCU were in the second group, those who recorded between 201 and 300 were in the third group, and so forth, until those few individuals who recorded between 600 and 1,000 units were in the highest LCU group. A positive, linear relationship was seen between magnitude of LCU scores for the previous year and the number of illnesses incurred during the overseas period.[20]

LCU Scores and the Immediacy of Illness

Extrapolating from retrospective findings, it appeared that the higher a subject's recent (six-month) LCU total, the "closer" he might be to future illness. To examine for evidence of such a relationship between LCU magnitude and immediacy of illness, first illnesses were considered separately. When first illnesses were tabulated for the men in LCU deciles 9 and 10 and compared with first illnesses for men in LCU deciles 1 and 2, the high LCU group (deciles 9 and 10) developed nearly twice as many first illnesses as the low LCU group during the first followup month; also, the high LCU group reported 60 percent more first illnesses during the second followup month. No significant differences were seen in first illness reporting between the high and low LCU groups for each of the remaining four months of the cruise. However, by this time the men most vulnerable to illness had already become ill.[12]

Relationships of LCU Scores to Illness Reports
by Age and Marital Status

Relationships of SRE questionnaire data to illness reports during overseas cruise periods were examined for more than 2,000 senior Navy enlisted men (petty officers) by age and marital status, categories.[9] (Similar analyses were done for junior enlisted men, but because of the restricted age range and predominantly single marital status, the sample was not well distributed along these demographic dimensions). For the entire sample of senior enlisted men, at least one illness was reported during the overseas period by about three fourths of the subjects. Deviations from this 75 percent general illness rate are shown in the various cells of Table IV-II for particular age and marital status subgroups. The Table is divided into quarters to facilitate interpretation of results. Older men (age 24 and above) who reported low amounts of life change (deciles 1 to 5) had illness rates well below the overall rate (—22%, —18%, —17% and —5%). In contrast, subgroups of younger men with higher life changes registered illness rates uniformly above the overall rate (+3% and +9%). Similarly, married men with low life change had relatively low illness rates (—15% and —11%), while single men with high life change had more illnesses than expected (+7% and +8%).

TABLE IV-II. DEVIATION OF ILLNESS RATES BY LCU
DECILES, AGE AND MARITAL STATUS*

Age (years):	LCU Deciles			
	1 and 2	*3 - 5*	*6 - 8*	*9 and 10*
Less than 22	—3%	—2%	+3%	+9%
	(N = 87)	(N = 168)	(N = 186)	(N = 112)
22-23	+7%	+7%	+6%	+6%
	(N = 52)	(N = 119)	(N = 119)	(N = 69)
24-29	—22%	—18%	+2%	+1%
	(N = 47)	(N = 88)	(N = 83)	(N = 71)
More than 29	—17%	—5%	+8%	—2%
	(N = 52)	(N = 78)	(N = 83)	(N = 34)
Marital Status:				
Single	—4%	+2%	+7%	+8%
	(N = 157)	(N = 268)	(N = 240)	(N = 77)
Married	—16%	—11%	+1%	+4%
	(N = 81)	(N = 183)	(N = 231)	(N = 209)

*Each cell's deviation from the overall 75 percent illness rate is indicated.

Specificity of Life Change Events for Particular Age and Marital Subgroups

Our Navy samples were predominantly unmarried males of a restricted age range (17 to 30 years, mean = 22 years). The kinds of recent life change events applicable to these young men (terminating school, residential moves, financial problems, troubles with superiors, traffic violations, etc.) generally resulted in low LCU values. Only when the enlisted men were older and married did they report events with relatively high LCU values such as marriage, birth of children, illness of family member, home mortgage and so forth. Hence, high LCU scores for young, single sailors were generally based upon numerous life changes with low LCU values while older, married enlisted men could achieve high LCU totals with only a few serious life changes. We found that the older, married men's cruise-period illness reports showed higher correlations with LCU scores than did the illness reports of the younger, single sailors.[18]

Specificity of life change events for particular age and marital status subgroups was examined by means of a series of regression analyses using enlisted subjects from the three cruisers. Generally, different life change events correlated with illness in the five age-marital subgroups studied. Three to five events proved to be rather specific for each particular subgroup. Recent disciplinary problems was the only life change category which tended to predict illness in more than one subgroup. A multiple correlation of o.36 was achieved for the older, married subgroup using five specific LCU items; the cross-validity coefficient for this equation, although significant, was only o.10, however.[18]

Cluster Analysis of Life Change Events

In an effort to aid conceptual definition and improve reliability of measurement, a cluster analysis of the forty-two SRE items was carried out, and twenty-four of the items were found to form four distinct and homogeneous clusters. Nine items comprised a personal and social events cluster, four items a work changes cluster, eight items a marital-family relations cluster, and three items a disciplinary cluster. The eighteen remaining life change items—many of them with very low frequencies of occurrence, such as divorce, death of a family member, etc.—tended to have low correlations with other life change events.[24]

Subjects in the cruiser sample were divided into subgroups based upon the numbers and combinations of cluster categories in which their life changes were distributed: no event in any cluster, one or more events in one cluster only (four categories), events in two of the four clusters (six categories), events in three clusters (four categories), or events in all four clusters. Subjects with recent life changes in the work, marital-family or personal-social clusters had progressively higher illness rates than subjects with no cluster events. Men with life changes exclusively in the disciplinary cluster category showed an illness rate of 40 percent greater than persons with no cluster events. The progressive increase in illness rate from the work cluster to the disciplinary cluster was roughly in accordance with the mean LCU values of the four clusters with the exception of LCU value for the personal-social cluster which was relatively low. The mean LCU values for the clusters were: work cluster—28, marital-family cluster—36, personal-social cluster—21 and disciplinary cluster—44.

Subjects with life events in multiple clusters tended to have more illnesses than subjects with events in a single cluster, except for those with events in the disciplinary cluster. Disciplinary events, whether alone or in combination with events from other clusters, appeared to have a marked effect upon illness rate. Also, the personal-social cluster seemed to have more effect than would be expected from the low LCU values of items in this cluster.

TABLE IV-III. ILLNESS RATES BY CLUSTER CATEGORIES AND COMBINATIONS OF CLUSTER CATEGORIES

Cluster Categories	No. of Cases	Illness Rate (No./1000 men/day)
No cluster events	280	7.3
(1) Work	211	7.5
(2) Marital-home	80	8.0
(3) Personal-social	255	8.4
(4) Disciplinary	31	10.1
(1) + (2)	144	7.5
(1) + (3)	511	9.2
(1) + (4)	27	12.2
(2) + (3)	143	8.4
(2) + (4)	11	12.0
(3) + (4)	47	14.6
(1) + (2) + (3)	534	8.2
(1) + (2) + (4)	10	8.0
(1) + (3) + (4)	93	12.8
(2) + (3) + (4)	18	9.6
(1) + (2) + (3) + (4)	90	12.2

Studies of Underwater Demolition Team (UDT) Trainees

A study of 247 UDT trainees attacked a particular problem in the SRE's ability to predict illness. Over three fourths of these UDT men were young, single, enlisted men—the group in which it had previously proven most difficult to predict near-future illness from recent life changes information. The following analysis involved 194 young, single UDT enlisted trainees. By paying special attention to the severities of illnesses these men reported, the subjects' SRE information was found to best predict relatively severe illnesses rather than minor ones.[14]

UDT training is an extremely stressful four-month training program described fully in a later chapter by Rubin and Rahe on UDT biochemical studies. Illness reports are extremely high during UDT training. For subjects who passed the course, the illness rate has been reported to be ten times higher than that for men aboard ship. For UDT subjects who dropped from training, and this percentage has ranged between 30 and 70 percent of the classes, the illness reporting rate has been seen to rise to fifty times that for shipboard subjects.[14]

The sample of 194 men was divided into two random halves in order to utilize a validation, cross-validation methodology. The list of forty-two life change events were correlated separately with subjects' illness reports in the first, or validation, half of the sample. Six life changes events were seen to have significant (all positive) correlations with the illness criterion. The multiple correlation of these six recent life events with subjects' illness reports in the validation sample was 0.42 ($p < 0.001$). In the cross-validation sample, an equation based on these six life changes correlated significantly, and in the predicted direction, with the cross-validation sample's illness reports (0.19; $p < 0.05$).

UDT trainees who drop from training do so in two ways. First, if they have performed well in training but develop relatively severe and/or disabling illnesses, they can be medically dropped from the program with a chance to be "recycled" into a subsequent UDT class. Second, if they are poor trainees who find they have insufficient motivation to cope with the stresses of training, they are "voluntarily" dropped from the course. It is usual, however, for voluntary drops to have developed some minor illnesses prior to their drop, often as a "save face" measure with peers and instructors. Medically and voluntarily dropped UDT subjects' SRE information (combining the validation and cross-validation samples) showed an overall correlation with the number of illness reports of 0.33 ($p < 0.01$). The correlation of SRE data with number of dispensary visits for medically dropped subjects (some of whom were medically disabled) was 0.50 ($p < 0.01$). The correlation of SRE data for voluntarily dropped subjects with the number of generally minor dispensary visits was 0.20 (nonsignificant).[14] Therefore, in dealing with young, single men engaged in strenuous training, where significant numbers of serious as well as minor illnesses and injuries occur, subjects' recent life changes information may best predict their severe medical illnesses.

The Royal Norwegian Navy Study: Cross-cultural Confirmation

A presentation to North Atlantic Treaty Organization (NATO) scientists in 1968 led to a cross-cultural replication study by two Norwegian Navy psychologists, Drs. Rolf Gerhardt and Ivar Fløistad. A Norwegian translation of the SRE was administered to more than 1,000 Norwegian enlisted sailors at the end of specialized training school, approximately three to six months after beginning active duty. Medical criterion data were gathered after these subjects completed their thirteen-month enlistments, and the records had been stored in a central repository. Two Norwegian physicians, Drs. Rastus Ringdahl and Thomas Bergen, collected and coded the medical data.[15]

Complete questionnaire and illness criterion data were obtained for 821 Norwegian sailors, and LCU scores, based upon life changes during the six months prior to recording of illnesses, were divided approximately into decile intervals. The mean illness rates (number of illnesses/1000 men/day) for the followup period are shown in Table IV-IV together with comparable data for the U. S. cruiser samples. It can be seen that Norwegian subjects in decile 1, all of whom claimed no recent life changes for the six months prior to the start of illness data collection, had the lowest illness rate (6.4 illnesses/1000 men/day). On the other hand, subjects in decile 10, men with 218 LCU or more during the six-month period prior to illness data collection, recorded a much higher illness rate (9.3 illnesses/1000 men/day).

Comparing the LCU score range for each of the deciles of the Norwegian Navy sample with that of the combined U. S. Navy cruiser sample, it was apparent that Norwegians reported less life change than did Americans. To further compare illness rates for the two samples, deciles were grouped according to LCU score intervals established for previous samples. In other words, for the American Navy sample the men in deciles 1 to 3 reported an LCU range of approximately 0 to 75 for the six months prior to the study (or 150 LCU units per year). In the Norwegian sample, subjects reporting 0 to 75 LCU per six-month period included deciles 1 to 5.

Life Stress and Illness

TABLE IV-IV. COMPARISON OF ILLNESS RATES FOR NORWEGIAN
AND U. S. SAMPLES BY LCU DECILES AND SCORE INTERVALS

Norwegian Sample

LCU Decile	No. of Cases	LCU Range (6 mos.)		Mean Ill- ness Rate
1	88	0		6.4
2	92	1–20		7.1
3	79	21–39	(0–75)*	7.2 (7.0)*
4	91	40–57		7.8
5	91	58–76		6.8
6	79	77–98		7.8
7	79	99–128	(76–150)	9.7 (8.2)
8	76	129–156		7.1
9	76	157–217		7.8
10	70	218+	(151–300)	9.3 (8.6)

U. S. Cruiser Sample

LCU Decile	No. of Cases	LCU Range (6 mos.)		Mean Ill- ness Rate
1	276	0–28		8.1
2	242	29–57	(0–75)	7.7 (7.7)
3	244	58–88		7.5
4	241	89–119	(76–150)	8.8 (8.5)
5	247	120–151		8.2
6	246	152–189		8.9
7	247	190–239	(151–300)	9.2 (9.2)
8	246	240–299		9.6
9	246	300–383	(300+)	9.5 (9.9)
10	250	384+		10.3

*Approximate LCU ranges and average illness rates are given in parentheses.

In the American sample, deciles 4 and 5 included subjects who
registered between 75 to 150 LCU over the prior six-month interval (or between 150 and 300 LCU per year), while in the Norwegian sample subjects with these scores were included in deciles
6 to 8. Only the American sample included any subjects with more
than 300 LCU for the six months prior to illness collection (deciles
9 and 10). It was interesting to note that when grouped by these
LCU intervals, the Norwegian and American samples reported
similar mean illness rates. The major difference between the samples
was that, group by group, the Norwegians reported fewer recent
life changes (and proportionately fewer illnesses) than did the
American subjects.

A Pearson product-moment correlation between six-month LCU scores and number of illnesses for the Norwegian Navy sample was 0.12 (p < 0.001). This correlation compared closely to that for the American Navy sample of 0.09 (p < 0.001).

DISCUSSION

The major purpose of the life changes and illness studies was to investigate the utility of the life changes method in predicting illness in various groups of subjects. Because most of the previous work done in this area had been retrospective in nature, complete assessment of the life changes method required prospective experimentation. Therefore, using shipboard samples, where illness data could be collected by medical personnel who did not know the subjects' LCU scores and did not know the research design, fulfilled the need for unbiased prospective work. It is important to emphasize, however, that our subjects were generally unmarried males around twenty-two years of age. The life changes reported by these men proved to be rather specific to their age, sex and marital status and the illnesses reported for these subjects were, by and large, minor in severity. Thus, these large-scale shipboard studies provided a prospective test of the predictive power of recent life changes with respect to minor illnesses. Despite these limitations, statistically significant relationships were shown between LCU scores and near-future illnesses. Moreover, these U. S. Navy findings have been replicated by other investigators in samples of flight officers, National Guard officer candidates and Norwegian Navy enlisted men.[1, 15, 25]

When large shipboard samples were broken down into subgroups by age and marital status categories, it was evident that the young, single sailor incurred a relatively high number of illness episodes. The older, married subjects generally had better health, but higher correlations were demonstrated between LCU scores and near-future illnesses in this group than in the younger, single group. This finding may have been partially due to the fact that married subjects could respond to several recent life change events in the SRE which were not applicable to the single sailors, thereby providing greater life changes variance for the married sailors.

The older, married subjects were a particularly interesting group in that when they reported low levels of pre-cruise life change, they subsequently incurred much less illness than did other married men with high LCU totals. It appeared, therefore, that an absence of recent life changes, especially for the older, married sailor, was an excellent predictor of health.

Several attempts were made to improve on the LCU scoring system. First, a stepwise regression analysis of the forty-two life changes identified nine life change events which added significantly and uniquely to the best predictive equation.[18] The multiple correlation coefficient was encouragingly high on the validation study, but cross-validation failed to sustain this relationship.[18] Because all significant recent life events determined by subsequent regression analyses proved to have *positive* correlations with the illness criterion and to have approximately equal LCU values, a unit scoring system was then utilized, particularly in the UDT studies. Finally, a cluster analysis of the forty-two life change events indicated the existence of four independent clusters among twenty-four of the life change items. A cluster scoring system, based on the data presented in Table IV-III, is currently being investigated. The best scoring systems for predicting near-future illnesses in various populations is still open to question and experimentation.

The Norwegian Navy cross-cultural study confirmed the results of both retrospective and prospective U. S. Navy studies. Both Norwegian and American Navy subjects reporting between 0 and 75 LCU for the six months prior to illness data collection incurred mean illness rates of slightly more than 7 illnesses/1000 men/day. The illness rate increased to approximately 8.5 illnesses/1000 men/ day for subjects with LCU values between 76 and 150 for the six months prior to study. Finally, those subjects with LCU totals between 151 and 300 registered nearly 9 illnesses/1000 men/day. Only the American sample had subjects with more than 300 LCU for the six months prior to follow-up: these men incurred 10 illnesses/1000 men/day.

When severity of illnesses was examined for the UDT trainees (a greater number of severe and disabling injuries and illnesses occurred in this group than in the shipboard samples) recent life changes significantly predicted the more serious illnesses but not the minor illnesses. Hence, it appeared that the illness criterion of our shipboard studies—minor illnesses—might not be the optimum criterion for testing the predictive validity of life changes.

Aside from the problem of minor illness as a criterion, the issue of symptom recognition, as a meaningful criterion, in addition to recorded illness, should be considered. In all of the foregoing studies, subjects were asked to report life changes for the previous six-month period and then illness data were collected during the following six months to one year. One may ask the question, "How many subjects actually perceived illness symptoms but failed to report them to the medical department?" In our studies we did ask all subjects to report their awareness of diffuse physical and psychological symptoms on the twenty-question Health Opinion Survey (HOS) questionnaire devised by Macmillan.[1] Therefore, relationships between life changes during the past six months and perception of body symptoms at the time of completing the questionnaires could be determined. This illness symptom criterion would have the advantage of being nearer in time to the life change events than the shipboard illness criterion data and perhaps represents a more immediate and direct response to life changes than later illness reports. For all U. S. Navy samples the correlation between LCU scores and HOS symptom scores was 0.32 (p < .001). For the Norwegian Navy sample this correlation was 0.23 (p < .001). These correlations between recent life changes and perceived symptoms are relatively high compared with correlations between life changes and illnesses as long as one year later (r approximately 0.10).

With the correlation between recent life changes and perceptions of bodily symptoms being higher than the correlation between life changes and near-future illnesses, one might reasonably ask, "What are the factors determining which subjects with symptoms report to the medical department and which subjects do not?" Illness rates have been shown to vary with age, education, occupation, job satisfaction, job status, race and marital status. Illness rate was seen to be positively associated with Negro race (less than 6% of crew), low job status and occupations which demanded the most arduous physical activity, and negatively related to age, education, job satisfaction and marital status (married). It seems clear that older, married men with better education and higher job satisfaction are much less likely to report minor illness symptoms to the medical department than younger, single individuals working in uncomfortable environments, experiencing numerous life changes, and perceiving bodily symptoms.

Subjects' recent life changes, perceptions of symptoms, and selected demographic, psychosocial and occupational characteristics appear to act in combination to precipitate illness episodes. To recapitulate this paper's Introduction, the importance of defining these precipitating factors is that such temporal factors may prove to be more readily brought under control than other predisposing factors, such as heredity. If this proves to be the case, the results will contribute to the ultimate aim of medicine—disease prevention.

REFERENCES

1. Cline, D.W., and Chosey, J.J.: A prospective study of life changes and subsequent health changes. *Arch Gen Psychiatr*, 27:51-53, 1972.
2. Gunderson, E.K.E., Rahe, R.H., and Arthur, R.J.: The epidemiology of illness in naval environments: II. Demographic, social background, and occupational factors. *Milit Med*, 135:453-458, 1970.
3. Hawkins, N.G., Davies, R., and Holmes, T.H.: Evidence of psychosocial factors in the development of pulmonary tuberculosis. *Am Rev Tuberc Pulmon Dis*, 75:5, 1957.
4. Hinkle, L.E., Jr., Redmont, R., Plummer, N., and Wolff, H.G.: An examination of the relation between symptoms, disability, and serious illness in two homogeneous groups of men and women. *Can J Public Health*, 50:1372, 1960.
5. Holmes, T.S., and Holmes, T.H.: Short-term intrusions into the life style routine. *J Psychosom Res*, 14:121, 1970.
6. Komaroff, A.L., Masuda, M., and Holmes, T.H.: The social readjustment rating scale. A comparative study of Negro, Mexican, and White Americans. *J Psychosom Res*, 12:21, 1968.
7. Macmillan, A.M.: The health opinion survey: Technique for estimating prevalence of psychoneurotic and related types of disorder in communities. *Psychol Rep*, 2:325, 1957.
8. Masuda, M., and Holmes, T.H.: The social readjustment rating scale. A cross-cultural study of Japanese and Americans. *J Psychosom Res*, 11:227, 1967.
9. Pugh, W., Gunderson, E.K.E., Erickson, J.M., Rahe, R.H., and Rubin, R.T.: Variations of illness incidence in the Navy population. *Milit Med*, 137:224-227, 1972.
10. Rahe, R.H.: Life crisis and health change. In May, Philip R.A., and Wittenborn, J.R. (Eds.): *Psychotropic Drug Response: Advances in Prediction*. Springfield, Ill., Thomas, 1969, pp. 92-125.
11. ————: Multi-cultural correlations of life change scaling: America, Japan, Denmark, and Sweden. *J Psychosom Res*, 13:191-195, 1969.

12. _____: Life change measurement as a predictor of illness. *Proc R Soc Med*, *61*:1124-1126, 1968.

13. ————, and Arthur, R.J.: Life changes surrounding illness experience. *J Psychosom Res*, *11*:341-345, 1968.

14. ————, Biersner, R.J., Ryman, D.H., and Arthur, R.J.: Psychosocial predictors of illness behavior and failure in stressful training. *J Health Soc Behav*, *13*:393-397, 1972.

15. ————, Fløistad, I., Bergen, T., Ringdahl, R., Gunderson, E.K.E., Gerhardt, R., and Arthur, R.J.: A comparative study of Norwegian Navy and American Navy subjects' life changes and illness onset. In press.

16. ————. Gunderson, E.K.E., and Arthur, R.J.: Demographic and psychosocial factors in acute illness reporting. *J Chronic Dis*, *23*:245-255, 1970.

17. ————, Gunderson, E.K.E., Pugh, W., Rubin, R.T., and Arthur, R.J.: Illness prediction studies. Use of psychosocial and occupational characteristics as predictors. *Arch Environ Health*, *25*:192-197, 1972.

18. ————, Jensen, P.D., and Gunderson, E.K.E.: Illness prediction by regression analysis of subjects' life changes information. *Unit Report 71-5*, U.S. Navy Medical Neuropsychiatric Research Unit, 1971.

19. ————, Lundberg, U., Bennett, L., and Theorell, T.: The social readjustment rating scale: A comparative study of Swedes and Americans. *J Psychosom Res*, *15*:241-249, 1971.

20. ————, Mahan, J., and Arthur, R.J.: Prediction of near-future health change from subjects' preceding life changes. *J Psychosom Res*, *14*:401-406, 1970.

21. ————, Mahan, J., Arthur, R.J., and Gunderson, E.K.E.: Epidemiology of illness in naval environments. I. Illness types, distribution, severities, and relationship to life change. *Milit Med*, *135*:443-452, 1970.

22. ————, McKean, J., and Arthur, R.J.: A longitudinal study of life change and illness patterns. *J Psychosom Res*, *10*:355-366, 1967.

23. ————, Meyer, H., Smith, M., Kjaer, G., and Holmes, T.H.: Social stress and illness onset. *J Psychosom Res*, *8*:35, 1964.

24. ————, Pugh, W.M., Erickson, J., Gunderson, E.K.E., and Rubin, R.T.: Cluster analysis of life changes, I. Consistency of clusters across large Navy samples. *Arch Gen Psychiatr*, *25*:332, 1971.

25. Rubin, R.T., Gunderson, E.K.E., and Arthur, R.J.: Life stress and illness patterns in the U.S. Navy, VI. Environmental, demographic, and prior life change variables in relation to illness onset in naval aviators during a combat cruise. *Psychosom Med*, *34*:533-547, 1972.

26. ————, Gunderson, E.K.E., and Arthur, R.J.: Life stress and illness patterns in the U.S. Navy, III. Prior life change and illness onset in an attack carrier's crew. *Arch Environ Health*, *19*:753-757, 1969.

27. Stevens, S.S.: A metric for the social consensus. *Science*, *151*:530, 1966.

28. Theorell, T., and Rahe, R.H.: Psychosocial factors and myocardial infarction. I. An inpatient study in Sweden. *J Psychosom Res*, *15*:25-31, 1971.

COMMENT

PAUL D. NELSON*

One familiar with the costs, and the pitfalls, inherent in the conduct of longitudinal studies of health and related behaviors must be impressed by the research on temporal factors in the prediction of illness by Rahe and his associates. Impressive, too, is the consistency in results relating frequency and magnitude of changes in an individual's life circumstances to the incidence and severity of illness. The basic thesis of this work, advanced earlier by such as Hinkle and Wolff,[15] is that certain life events can be ordered with respect to the extent to which they are potentially threatening, disruptive or require readjustment in the individual's mode of life. Further, it is hypothesized that the intensity or magnitude of threat, disruption or readjustment evoked by such life events is associated with emotional arousal and neuroendocrine changes which, if prolonged, may result in impaired functioning or illness.

Kagan has argued that the causal link between psychosocial stressors, stress and disease must be regarded as speculative until better conceptualization and measurement of pertinent variables can be achieved by means of experimental epidemiological studies.[17] The research described by Rahe is a step in the direction advocated by Kagan for one type of psychosocial stressors, namely, life change events.

It is perhaps frustrating to Rahe and his colleagues that life change scores obtained from the *Schedule of Recent Experience* thus far have only low correlations with illness incidence among young Navy enlisted men. Other variables, such as age, job specialty, work environment, illness history and job satisfaction, correlate as highly as life change scores with dispensary visits aboard ship. However,

*Commander, Medical Service Corps, U. S. Navy

this fact does not diminish the importance of determining the significance of life change events for future illness in a variety of populations and settings. Improvements in measurement techniques, identification of high risk populations, and the use of multiple regression methods should enhance the prognostic significance of life change measures in selected groups and situations.

Observations of illness patterns aboard several types of ships by Rahe and his colleagues,[31, 34, 36] normative studies of psychosomatic symptoms by Gunderson et al.,[14] and longitudinal studies of health and behavior problems among first-enlistment sailors by Plag et al.[25, 26] indicate that a rather small proportion of men account for a large proportion of sick days lost. These men tend to be immature and less capable individuals who occupy the more routine jobs requiring less skill, often in the more hazardous or uncomfortable areas of the ship. One might wonder whether the "sick role," as characterized by the American sociologist Talcott Parsons,[24] might not be a way of coping with situational pressures for some of these sailors. The illnesses recorded by Rahe and his associates were only those that actually required treatment, however, and not simply the ill-defined complaints of malingerers. Because dermatological problems were among the most prevalent illnesses recorded,[34] one still might ask about the prevalence of minor rashes, skin infections, burns, etc., among sailors who did not appear at the dispensary for treatment but remained on the job. A related question which might be answered easily is: What are the characteristics of sailors who report for minor medical care by self-referral as opposed to those who are referred by superiors?

From my interpretation of Rahe's data, the sailors most likely to report frequent or important life changes are married men with children who have had a recent illness and are concerned about their health as evidenced by psychosomatic complaints. The key variable in this cluster might be the recent illness. As Rahe has reported elsewhere,[29] life changes tend to cluster subsequent to illness as well as prior to it. Among sailors who are in the process of recovering from and adapting to the effects of an illness or injury, especially with the burden of family responsibilities and recent separation from family by returning to sea, which individuals are most likely to relapse or have further medical problems at sea? This question would seem to be an important one which has not been addressed by Rahe's data. It seems plausible that recovery and readjustment might be impeded or further health problems incurred by those who experience many life changes after a recent illness.

As Levi[21] has indicated in his conceptual model of psychosocial stresses and disease, many variables interact with recent life stresses to determine health changes and influence outcomes. One set of variables which cannot be ignored would be individual differences in social status and roles, personality traits, value systems, cultural life styles and aspirations as well as past successes and failure. Such patterns of individual characteristics need to be better defined and their relationships to the impact of stressful life change events determined in order to assess their significance for health and adaptation. The perceptual-cognitive emphasis given by Lazarus[19,20] in his discussion of stress and emotion is an essential part of any conceptualization of life events as stressors whether or not such stressors result in illness. Cognitive processes influence what we attend to, how we interpret the significance of events in context, how we respond emotionally, how we behave in coping with life events, and, indeed, how we evaluate our success or failure in coping with stress.

It was largely on this basis that Holmes and Rahe[16] developed the *Social Readjustment Rating Questionnaire* and the *Schedule of Recent Experience*. Drawing from a wide sampling of life events and behavior changes presented in interview material, items were scaled by the method of constant stimuli, using marriage as the constant stimulus against which other life events could be compared. The perceptual-cognitive processes inherent in these psychophysical scaling procedures have been shown to yield highly similar judgments across individuals and groups.[8,39]

To determine the extent to which the selected set of life change items have comparable scale values across different populations, Rahe and his colleagues have repeated the life scaling procedures on an assortment of samples varying in age, sex, ethnic and socioeconomic backgrounds. The hope was to develop a standard metric which in a nomothetic model would be generalizable over individuals and across different cultural groups. Variations were observed between certain samples in the relative significance assigned to selected life change items, such as the much greater significance attributed to a jail term by a sample of middle-class Americans of Caucasian background in contrast to a lower socioeconomic group of Mexican-Americans or the reverse in relation to taking a mortgage of over ten thousand dollars. Interesting too are variations suggesting that Swedes generally give higher scale values to life change items than do Americans, and older Swedish citizens generally higher values than younger, perhaps suggesting greater stability in the Swedish way of life and greater impact of variations, particularly among the older citizens.

The generally high correlations in mean scale values for different life change events across various samples have nevertheless led to the conclusion that the *Schedule of Recent Experience* life change items have general significance for different groups. It seems plausible that among Western societies and those within their cultural influence there are general norms and values associated with such matters as birth and death, health and illness, family relations, friendships, work and social behavior, and people are able to make judgments about the relative importance of such matters in a general way whether they have experienced them or not. The late Hadley Cantril,[4] in his cross-national study of the hopes, fears, concerns and aspirations of people from many stations in life in older established and newly emerging societies, similarly noted common patterns of value orientation among diverse peoples, apparently because they are human.

But the variation in significance of life change items about group mean scale values—certainly present in Rahe's cross-cultural studies as in Cantril's—cannot be altogether ignored if one is to relate life events and their interpretations by individuals to stress states and even, perhaps, to health change. While, indeed, there may be some common orientations among different peoples about the general significance of such events as death in a family, marriage, a jail term or a change in one's job, the perceived significance and evoked emotional, physiological and behavioral coping patterns are likely to vary as a function of personal characteristics of the individual and the context of life experience in which they occur.

The impact of life events upon the individual can vary as a function of the intensity and magnitude with which events are perceived to vary from preceding stimulus states or normal activity baselines,[7,10,37] the suddenness or unpredictability with which an event occurs,[5] or, conversely, the degree of preparedness of the individual by virtue of previous experience or anticipation of an event.[6,19] Inability to make a monthly rental payment to the landlord undoubtedly has a different impact upon one who has always made such payments in a timely manner as contrasted to one whose inability to do so has become a monthly routine; or, as the American television host Johnny Carson once put it, having a sex change operation is traumatic enough, but discovering one has had a sex change operation after going into surgery for a tonsillectomy is an event of life crisis proportions!

Then, too, man is not simply a passive spectator of environmental events; he has the capacity and often the inclination to act upon his environment in such a way as to create change or bring about what we have referred to as life changes. The studies of Rosenman et al., which focused upon personality types in relation to coronary heart disease, suggested the importance of aggressive versus passive orientations toward one's environment as a factor in illness incidence.[33] One's role in a particular setting, the individual's perception of the expectations held of him by others, and his perceived ability to control or alter a situation, are important factors in understanding how life events are interpreted and what reactions and coping mechanisms are evoked. Rubin's study of biochemical patterns differentiating pilots from their radar intercept operators during aircraft carrier landings,[35] Peter Bourne's excellent and unusual study of Special Forces officers and NCO's in preparation for and under attack in combat,[1] and, of course, Brady's classical "excutive monkey" study[2] illustrate the importance of interpersonal roles and related perceptual-cognitive processes in the interpretation and subsequent reaction to stressful life events.

I also wonder about the possible differences among individuals in the relative frequency with which certain types of life change events have characterized their lives, regardless of their need for change or other personality traits. Is the individual's ability to withstand or cope with life changes during adult years at all affected by prior frequent change in life circumstances, for example, frequency of family moves, or changes in living habits consequent to changes in employment or income?

While frequency of life change is important in the scheme of things to Rahe and his colleagues, the significance of magnitude or intensity of life change events, in terms of subsequent adjustment required, is more central to their conceptualization of life change in relation to stress and health. That being the case, more attention might be given in the life change questionnaire measurement system to the importance of the following: the situational context in which life events have occurred, including the individual's role in these events; the extent to which these life changes were a function of the individual's own behavior and the extent to which his personal responsibilities were altered as a function of the change; the related matter of whether those events were anticipated, that is, how prepared the individual was for them, or perhaps the amount of experience previously gained from similar types of change earlier; and those characteristics of personality, personal and cultural values, and aspirations which might influence the way in which an individual interprets and copes with such life changes. Attempts to evaluate the predictive validity of life changes for health status in different age, occupational or demographic subgroups is a step in the proper direction, but many more variables need to be assessed, some of which may require modification of the life change questionnaire itself (for example, getting at the context in which the life event occurred).

It is in regard to coping with life events, a matter to which Lazarus[19] has suggested more attention be given in our conceptualization of stress, that the *Schedule of Recent Experience Questionnaire* might especially be reevaluated. Some of the life change items, for example, change in one's personal habits, perhaps even such items as marriage or divorce, might for many individuals reflect an active coping with or adjustment to another life event or series of life events, effective for some and not for others. Other items, such as death of spouse, are not, of course, of the same nature. How an individual attempts to cope with life events requiring readjustment, as well as his perception of success or failure in that endeavor, should be assessed, difficult as that task might be.

The focus of attention among Rahe's colleagues at present appears to be the psychometric properties of the *Schedule of Recent Experience Questionnaire* as indicated by recent cluster analyses of life change items[22] and reliability studies of life change cluster scores,[23] as well as the addition of new items of life change significance and the simplification of current items.

The emphasis also being given by Rahe and his associates to the work environment, job attitudes and occupational culture of various groups of naval personnel provides an important context for better understanding the significance of life change events for sailors, as well as the coping process related to such changes, in relation to physical and mental health. Gardell's analysis[12] of mental health among industrial workers having different levels of job complexity, feelings of competence, involvement in organizational planning and perceived value of one's work relative to personal levels of aspiration—a study discussed in the Stockholm symposium on stress and disease two years ago—suggests a number of hypotheses which might be pursued in studies aboard ship. The possible importance of work group cohesion as a moderating influence for the individual stressed by personal life circumstances,[13] or perhaps the aggravating conditions of role conflict or role ambiguity on the job,[18] suggest still further dimensions of one's work environment which might serve as moderator variables in the link between life changes outside the job and one's health. Indeed, such variables may be the primary sources of stress themselves, especially for those whose job, occupation or work organization constitutes a predominant role in the individual's total life space, a major source of personal gratification.

To summarize, the assessment of frequency and psychological magnitude of changes in one's life circumstances or personal habits, presumed to be stressors to the extent that some state of disequilibrium is evoked and readjustment required of the individual, is a start in the direction of better defining and measuring those personal-environmental variables which, at least theoretically, are predictors of stress and perhaps illness. But the moderator variables are many and demand attention, too. It is difficult to conceive of an adequate theory of stress which does not in some way involve the psychological elements of perception and cognition; and, those elements in turn would seem to require that attention be given to the environmental context or the event structure within which life changes occur as well as attributes of the individual's roles, personality, culture, past experience, aspirations, and his physical and mental states of health as they may relate to such life changes, their interpretation, and the emotional, physiological and behavioral responses which may be evoked. Complex multivariate models of analysis are clearly called for.

Complicating that requirement is the fact that many of the moderator variables in which we are interested are at the same time in an equivocal conceptual and metric state, the taxonomic ordering of environment and personality being examples.[9,10,38] Frederiksen,[11] who in a recent issue of the *American Psychologist* addressed the complexity of such issues, summarized the relative merits of various multivariate analytic techniques such as discriminant and factor analyses and offered the work of Tucker[40] and Levin[22] on multimode factor analysis as promising in our pursuit of more definitive dimensions of person-environment transactions. Response factors, situation factors, and person factors were extracted by Levin and Tucker in a study of reaction to different types of situations presumed to be of varying degrees and qualities of stressfulness. The concept of multitrait-multimethod analysis advanced by Campbell and Fiske,[3] recently explicated by Fiske[9] in his book on the concepts and measurement of personality, appears similarly of potential value to the assessment of stressors, stress and consequent adaptation or maladaptation.

Perhaps through our common orientations, though different approaches, to the general problem of stress and health, we might come to better understand those other constructs of person-environment transactions which have been so elusive for so long. Meanwhile, from a practical point of view, the research of Rahe and his colleagues, as that of others at this symposium, is highly important for its descriptive epidemiological value in advancing our awareness, understanding and prediction of health change within work environments of civilian and military communities alike.

REFERENCES

1. Bourne, Peter G., Rose, Robert M., and Mason, John W.: 17-OHCS levels in combat, Special Forces "A" Team under threat of attack. *Arch Gen Psychiatr, 19*:135-145, 1968.
2. Brady, J.V.: Ulcers in "executive" monkeys, *Sci Am, 199*:95-100, 1958.
3. Campbell, D.T., and Fiske, D.W.: Convergent and discriminant validi-

ties by the multitrait-multimethod matrix. *Psychol Bull,* 56:81-195, 1959.
4. Cantril, H.: *The Pattern of Human Concerns.* New Brunswick, N.J., Rutgers University Press, 1965.
5. Carlestam, G., and Levi, L.: *Urban Conglomerates as Psychosocial Human Medical Implications.* Sweden, Royal Ministry for Foreign Affairs and Royal Ministry of Agriculture, 1971.
6. Bassell, John: Physical illness in response to stress. In Levine, Sol, and Scotch, Norman A. (Eds.): *Social Stress.* Chicago, Aldine Publishing Co., 1970.
7. Dohrenwend, Barbara S., and Dohrenwend, Bruce P.: Class and race as status related sources of stress. In Levine, Sol, and Scotch, Norman A. (Eds.): *Social Stress.* Chicago, Aldine Publishing Co., 1970.
8. Ekman, Gosta: The measurement of subjective reaction. In Levi, L. (Ed.): *Emotional Stress.* Stockholm, Forsvarmedicin, 1967, Vol. 3, Suppl. 2.
9. Fiske, D.W.: *Measuring the Concepts of Personality.* Chicago, Aldine Publishing Co., 1971.
10. ———, and Maddi, S.R.: *Functions of Varied Experience.* Homewood, Ill., The Dorsey Press, Inc., 1961.
11. Frederiksen, Norman: Toward a taxonomy of situations. *Am Psychol,* 27:114-124, 1972.
12. Gardell, Bertil: Alienation and mental health in the modern industrial environment. In Levi, L. (Ed.): *Society, Stress and Disease.* London, Oxford University Press, 1971.
13. Gross, Edward: Work, organization, and stress. In Levine, Sol, and Scotch, Norman A. (Eds.): *Social Stress.* Chicago, Aldine Publishing Co., 1970.
14. Gunderson, E.K. Eric, Arthur, Ransom J., and Wilkins, Walter L.: A mental health survey instrument: The Health Opinion Survey. *Milit Med, 133:*306-311, 1968.
15. Hinkle, L.E., and Wolff, H.M.: The nature of man's adaptation to his total environment and the relation of this to illness. *Arch Intern Med, 99:*442-460, 1957.
16. Holmes, T.H., and Rahe, R.H.: The social readjustment rating scale. *J Psychosom Res, 11:*213, 1967.
17. Kagan, Aubrey: Epidemiology and society, stress and disease. In Levi, L. (Ed.): *Society, Stress, and Disease.* London, Oxford University Press, 1971.
18. Kahn, R.L., Wolfe, D.M., Quinn, R., Snock, J.D., and Rosenthal, R.A.: *Organizational Stress: Studies in Role Conflict and Ambiguity.* New York, John Wiley, 1961.
19. Lazarus, Richard S.: Cognitive and personality factors underlying threat and coping. In Levine, Sol, and Scotch, Norman A. (Eds.): *Social Stress.* Chicago, Aldine Publishing Co., 1970.

20. _____, Averill, James R., and Opton, Edward M.: Towards a cognitive theory of emotion. In Levi, L. (Ed.): *Society, Stress, and Disease*. London, Oxford University Press, 1971.

21. Levi, L.: The psychosocial environment and psychomatic disease. In Levi, L. (Ed.): *Society, Stress, and Disease*. London, Oxford University Press, 1971, vol. 1.

22. Levin, J.: Three-mode factor analysis. *Psychol Bull, 64*:442-452, 1965.

23. McDonald, B.W., Pugh, W.M., Gunderson, E.K.E., and Rahe, R.H.: Reliability of life change cluster scores. *Br J Soc Clin Psychol, 2*: 407-409, 1972.

24. Parsons, Talcott: Illness and the role of the physician: A sociological perspective. *Am J Orthopsychiatr, 21*:452-460, 1951.

25. Plag, John A., and Phelan, James D.: The epidemiology of illness among first-term naval enlistees. I. Incidence by type of illness and length of service. *Am J Epidemiol, 92*:1-12, 1970.

26. _____, Arthur, Ransom J., and Goffman, Jerry M.: Dimensions of psychiatric illness among first-term enlistees in the United States Navy. *Milit Med, 135*:665-673, 1970.

27. Pugh, W.M., Gunderson, E.K.E., Erickson, J.M., Rahe, R.H., and Rubin, R.T.: Variations of illness in the Navy population. *Milit Med, 137*:224-227, 1972.

28. Rahe, Richard H.: Multi-cultural correlations of life change scaling: America, Japan, Denmark and Sweden. *J. Psychosom Res, 13*:191-195, 1969.

29. _____: Life crisis and health change. In May, P.R.A. and Wittenborn, J.R. (Eds.): *Psychotropic Drug Response: Advances in Prediction*. Springfield, Ill., Thomas, 1969.

30. _____, Lundberg, U., Bennett, L., and Theorell, T.: The social readjustment rating scale: A comparative study of Swedes and Americans. *J Psychosom Res, 15*:241-249, 1971.

31. _____, Mahan, Jack L., Arthur, Ransom J., and Gunderson, E.K.E.: The epidemiology of illness in naval environments. I. Illness types, distribution, severities, and relationship of life change. *Milit Med, 135*:442-452, 1970.

32. _____, Pugh, W.M., Erickson, J.M., Gunderson, E.K.E., and Rubin, R.T.: Cluster analyses of life change: I. Consistency of clusters across large Navy samples. *Arch Gen Psychiatr, 25*:330-332, 1971.

33. Rosenman, R.H., Friedman, M., Straus, R., Wurm, M., Jenkins, C.D., and Messenger, M.B.: Coronary heart disease in the Western collaborative study group. *JAMA, 195*:86-92, 1966.

34. Rubin, Robert T., Gunderson, E.K.E., and Doll, Richard E.: Life stress and illness patterns in the U.S. Navy: I. Environmental variables and illness onset in an attack carrier's crew. *Arch Environ Health, 18*: 740-747, 1969.

35. ————, Miller, R.C., Arthur, R.J., and Clark, B.R.: Differential adreno-cortical stress responses among Navy pilots and their flight officers during aircraft carrier landing practice. *Psychol Rep, 25*:71-74, 1970.

36. ————, Gunderson, E.K.E., and Arthur, R.J.: Life stress and illness patterns in the U.S. Navy: IV. Environmental and demographic vari-ables in relation to illness onset in a battleship's crew. *J Psychosom Res, 15*:277-288, 1971.

37. Scott, Robert, and Howard, Alan: Models of stress. In Levine, Sol, and Scotch, Norman A. (Eds.): *Social Stress*. Chicago, Aldine Publish-ing Co., 1970.

38. Sells, S.B.: An interactionist looks at the environment. *Am Psychol, 18*: 696-702, 1963.

39. Stevens, S.S.: A metric for the social consensus. *Science, 151*:530-541, 1966.

40. Tucker, L.R.: Some mathematical notes on three-mode factor analysis. *Psychometrika, 31*:279-311, 1966.

Chapter V

PSYCHOSOCIAL CHARACTERISTICS OF SUBJECTS WITH MYOCARDIAL INFARCTION IN STOCKHOLM

Töres Theorell and Richard H. Rahe

INTRODUCTION

THE FOLLOWING represents a brief review of studies of psychological factors related to myocardial infarction (MI). MI subjects have been noted to prominently display personality traits such as aggressiveness, explosiveness and hostility.[11-13, 34] Dissatisfaction with their lives in general, especially with their work and their perceived lack of achievement at work, are common feelings and perceptions of MI subjects.[22, 25, 32, 34, 40, 42] Subjects developing MI notably work long hours, including substantial overtime work.[8, 19, 22, 32] Such a heavy investment in their work, often at the expense of their family lives, has led some authors to label these subjects "work addicts."[40] Men developing MI have also been noted to have a higher than expected incidence of psychiatric disturbances, including sexual difficulties and complaints of physical exhaustion.[22, 41] Psychoanalytically oriented authors have commented upon MI subjects' conflicts with a dominant father figure.[4] In addition, others have raised the question whether the MI subjects' aggressive achievement behavior is really a reaction formation to a feminine identification.[9, 14]

Studies which have focused upon social characteristics of MI victims include the following. During the early part of the twentieth century, myocardial infarction was seen (in England and America) to be primarily a disease of persons in the upper social classes. Nowadays, such a trend does not appear to exist and, if anything, atherosclerotic heart disease is more common in lower class subjects.[3] Among middle class men, MI seems to be slightly more common among those who hold foreman or supervisory positions.[3] It has been reported that subjects who have several changes of job and/or residence over the past few years have a higher incidence of MI than more stable subjects.[35] High school educated men competing for jobs with college educated men show higher MI rates at all age levels than the college men in one large company.[17] Finally, a study of a small community of Italian-Americans found that the men in this community had extremely low incidence and prevalence rates for MI, especially in the younger age groups. From a sociological viewpoint, these men formed a solid social community characterized by interpersonal warmth, stability and mutual interdependence. These lower MI rates, as well as these sociological features, were in contrast to relatives of these men living in neighboring U. S. communities.[7]

Psychological and social characteristics of MI subjects have been inferred primarily from retrospective studies of subjects who had already developed MI.[23,36] However, such information has also been obtained from prospective studies of healthy subjects who went on to develop MI. Psychological and social characteristics found of significance in prospective studies have included the following. A behavior pattern referred to as "Type A," primarily composed of hard-driving, competitive and time-urgent pursuits, has proven to be a significant predictor of MI.[29] Inordinate emphasis on work, rather than family life, as well as ambivalent feelings toward members of the same sex, have been cited by some to be predictive of MI.[5] Dissatisfaction with one's work and with one's marital life (seen as lack of emotional support from one's spouse) has been recently demonstrated to be predictive of MI in a large follow-up study in Israel.[24] Status incongruity, as measured by a discrepancy between parents' levels of education (and occupation), has been reported as a social characteristic predictive of subsequent MI.[33] Finally, subjects with relatively little formal education, as compared to others with whom they work, were more apt to develop MI in a longitudinal study carried out in Gothenburg, Sweden.[2]

A word should be said regarding a major qualitative difference between certain of the above-mentioned social and psychological characteristics of subjects prone to develop MI. That is, some of these factors represent *predisposing* characteristics of subjects who develop MI. Other psychological and social factors represent *precipitating* factors of MI onset. Certainly life-long behavior patterns, early childhood experiences and educational level have to be seen as long-standing "predisposing factors" to development of MI. These factors might be compared to predisposing "physical risk factors," such as blood pressure or serum cholesterol.[20] "Precipitating factors," however, include events like death of spouse.[26] Residential moves, recent promotions, recent changes in workload, recent change in marital status, and so forth, have been shown to be important precipitating factors in MI.[21, 27, 28, 36, 38]

Whether or not the above-mentioned psychological and social characteristics of subjects ultimately prove to be of etiologic importance in the onset of myocardial infarction, such information has already been seen to be extremely important in the rehabilitation of MI survivors. Several studies have shown that the spouse's attitude toward the patient, his socioeconomic class, his level of education and his behavior regarding his work and home life are extremely important in the adjustment he makes following MI.[16, 18, 30, 31, 37]

STOCKHOLM STUDIES
Retrospective Investigations

A retrospective study of social factors of importance in MI was carried out at the Seraphimer Hospital, Stockholm, using interviews (by a social worker) of 106 consecutive survivors of MI between the ages of forty and fifty-nine years. These MI survivors were compared with age-matched controls currently living in the same Stockholm area. Of statistical significance were the following: Patients tended to have come from larger families, to have had less formal education, to have been more frequently found unfit for military service, and to currently work longer hours per week than control subjects. (Infarction patients included several individuals who worked more than 60 hours per week whereas in Sweden the average work week is 42.5 hours.) Additionally, MI survivors reported more conflicts with teachers in school and with supervisors at work than did comparison subjects. The above differences were found to be more accentuated for males forty to forty-nine years of age than for men fifty to fifty-nine years old.[23]

A second study consisted of a sample of 62 male MI survivors who were sent a brief, self-administered behavior questionnaire. Questions asked covered the year prior to the onset of infarction, and responses were compared to answers for a group of 109 males of similar age who had no history of coronary heart disease (CHD) upon recent physical examination. Statistically significant differences between the MI survivors and the comparison group included the following: MI survivors reported more overtime work; they felt more dissatisfaction with their working conditions and with their lack of advancement at work than did comparison subjects; comparison subjects admitted to greater responsibility at work, more dissatisfaction with their levels of income, and more outside interests and activities, including physical activity, than did the MI survivors.[37]

Several small retrospective investigations into precipitating factors of MI were carried out at the Seraphimer Hospital. The first study consisted of 54 consecutive male survivors of MI admitted to one of the medical wards at the hospital in 1967 and 1968. A comparison sample included 14 close friends of these infarction patients, examined and found free of heart disease at the time of hospital visits to the patients.[36] A third group consisted of 30 male patients who had survived MI's for three to five years and continued to return to the Outpatient Department.[28] Finally, data from the spouses of 39 subjects who had died suddenly from their coronary heart disease were gathered.[27] All groups were requested to complete the Schedule of Recent Experience life changes questionnaire. The spouses of the sudden death group were requested to complete the questionnaire as it applied to their deceased mates. This questionnaire, along with the scaling method for the life change questions in terms of Life Change Units (LCU), has been outlined in a previous chapter in this volume by Rahe.

Survivors of MI, whether the MI occurred recently or years ago, demonstrated significantly elevated LCU levels during the six months *prior to* their infarctions (Figs. V-1 and V-2). Healthy friends of the recent infarction patients showed no LCU elevations in their own lives for the same six-month period that the MI group revealed significant elevations. Finally, spouses of sudden death victims reported

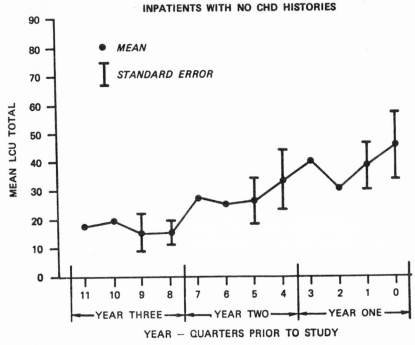

Figure V-1. LCU build-up over 3 years prior to MI for subjects with no prior history for CHD.

significantly elevated LCU levels for their deceased mates in the six months immediately prior to death (Fig. V-3). These findings have been replicated in larger samples, and the significance of these results is amplified in the chapter in this volume by Rahe and Romo.

Prospective Investigations

A group of 21 male subjects, aged forty-five to sixty-six years, who had survived an MI and had returned to their pre-infarction daily lives, were closely followed over a three-month period. Each subject was urged to remain on a standard diet and to keep his physical activity as well as his consumption of drugs, alcohol and tobacco as constant as possible. Subjects appeared in clinic weekly, whereupon they were evaluated for their current cardiovascular status and interviewed, utilizing the Schedule of Recent Experience questionnaire, for life changes experienced over the previous seven days. Results from this study showed a significant intrasubject co-

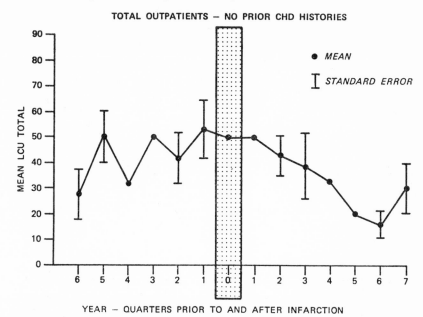

TOTAL OUTPATIENTS – NO PRIOR CHD HISTORIES

YEAR – QUARTERS PRIOR TO AND AFTER INFARCTION

Figure V-2. LCU build-up and fall-off prior to and following MI. Time of MI indicated by dotted column. All subjects were outpatients who had experienced a MI 3 to 5 years previously as their first symptom of CHD.

variation between their twelve-hour (daytime) urinary epinephrine output for the day prior to their clinic visit and their LCU total for the week prior to their visit ($r = 0.32$, $p < 0.001$). A statistically significant, but less striking, intrasubject covariation was also seen between subjects' weekly LCU totals and their daytime urinary norepinephrine output for the day prior to clinic visit ($r = 0.21$, $p < 0.05$). A full picture of correlations between weekly LCU totals and several biochemical dimensions (urinary epinephrine and norepinephrine, serum cholesterol, serum triglycerides, serum uric acid and serum creatinine), along with selected intercorrelations among these variables, is presented in Table V-I. Not all subjects showed a positive correlation between weekly LCU total and daytime epinephrine output, but six subjects demonstrated correlations greater than 0.70 between these two measures. (See Table V-II.)

Weekly LCU totals and complete physiological data for two subjects are graphically presented in Figures V-4 and V-5. Summaries of their weekly life changes are given below.

Life Stress and Illness

ALL SUDDEN DEATH SUBJECTS

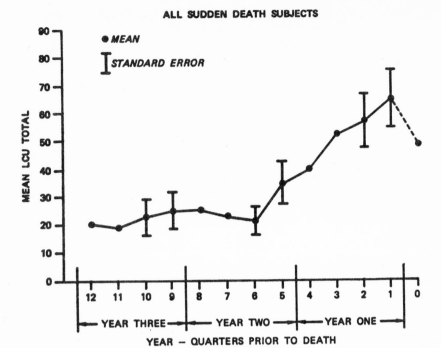

Figure V-3. LCU build-up (as recorded by next of kin) for subjects dying suddenly from their CHD.

TABLE V-I. INTRA-SUBJECT CORRELATIONS BETWEEN WEEKLY LIFE CHANGE UNIT (LCU) TOTALS AND PHYSIOLOGICAL VALUES FOR THE LAST DAY OF THE WEEK

(No. of cases = 130 to 147)

	LCU/week	Epinephrine daytime output	Norepinephrine daytime output
Epinephrine daytime output	0.32*		
Norepinephrine daytime output	0.21†	0.72*	
Serum cholesterol	0.06	—0.07	—0.05
Serum triglyceride	—0.15	—0.08	—0.09
Serum uric acid	—0.02	0.17†	0.23‡
Serum creatinine	0.16	0.03	0.10

*$p < 0.001$
†$p < 0.05$
‡$p < 0.01$

TABLE V-II INTRA-INDIVIDUAL PRODUCT MOMENT CORRELATIONS
(r) BETWEEN LIFE CHANGE TOTALS/WEEK AND
EPINEPHRINE (DAY) OUTPUT

Case No.	No. of Observations	r
1	9	0.87
2	7	0.85
3	6	0.84
4	7	0.84
5	6	0.74
6	9	0.71
7	7	0.60
8	7	0.43
9	4	0.41
10	8	0.35
11	7	0.34
12	3	0.24
13	8	0.19
14	14	0.14
15	10	0.12
16	4	0.07
17	9	0.01
18	8	—0.29
19	9	—0.37
20	6	—0.42

Subject 1 was a married foreman in an industrial firm with two sons still living at home. The first week of his follow-up he reported arguments at home and some new personnel at work which resulted in frustrations for him. Furthermore, his wife had just stopped working. The patient reported some apprehensiveness regarding his heart condition after reading a newspaper article on sudden cardiac death. The second week the subject reported arguments with his boss following a day off work. The third week the patient's mother was discovered to be seriously ill with cancer. During week four he reported that he had taken further days off work. Also, another relative had died suddenly. During the fifth week, further arguments with the subject's boss were reported over his work absences. Week six found the subject having to take days off work again due to new health problems in the family. Week seven, the subject reported a close friend had had a MI; in addition, he had visited relatives over the weekend. During week eight, the patient's mother had to be taken to the hospital, requiring him to take more time from work. During the ninth week the subject's mother was operated upon and during that week he also reported arguments with his wife over her health. During the tenth week, further arguments arose in the family, and he developed further worries regarding his mother's health. His frequent absences from work led to continuing arguments with his boss. His wife began and then stopped a new job during the same week. During the twelfth week she found a new job. The subject's urinary epinephrine output hit peaks during weeks four and eight—when a close relative had died, and when his mother was taken to the hospital. He also reported angina pectoris to the doctor when he learned his mother had cancer and when she had her operation.

Subject 2 was a 60-year-old part-time social worker and part-time journalist who was married with three sons still living at home. He had a previous MI in 1963 and a second MI in 1967. During his first follow-up week the subject reported he was involved in social work problems with immigrants to Sweden, and, although his work was

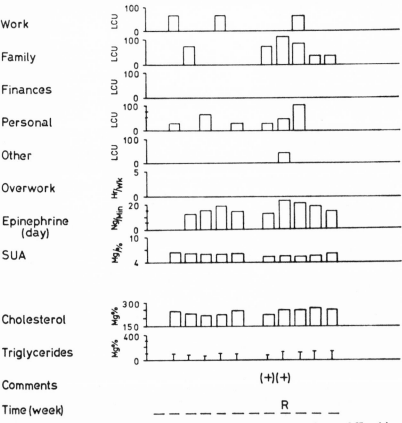

Figure V-4. Life changes and biochemical data for a second post-MI subject followed weekly over a 3-month interval.

going successfully, he was working quite a bit overtime. He reported some arguments with a son at home and also he had just received a parking ticket. During the second follow-up week he had guests in his home and also had to work a good deal overtime. Week four was notable in that the subject had flown to London the previous week and had been appointed as chairman of an European society dealing with his particular specialty in social work. His epinephrine output this fourth week was the highest of the follow-up period. His wife also began some academic studies that week. Week five he took one day off work for vacation and made some minor purchases. Week six found the subject slightly depressed over some arguments with his wife. Week eight the subject's boss had suddenly become seriously ill which meant more work for the subject. During the ninth week he continued to worry over the health of his boss and the amount of

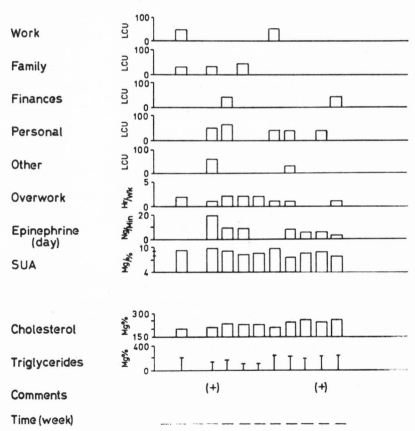

Figure V-5. Life changes and biochemical data for one post-MI subject followed weekly over a 3-month interval.

work he had plus important visitors coming to the country. During week eleven he reported worries about his health. His serum cholesterol and triglycerides both reached their highest levels during these later weeks of the follow-up interval. During week twelve he purchased a new automobile. This subject was one of several men in this study who showed correlations between serum cholesterol and triglycerides with a reported sense of worry and feelings of depression. He had a high and slightly variable serum uric acid output throughout the entire follow-up period. Reports of angina pectoris were given in week four when he had recently been elected chairman of the European Society and during week eleven when he expressed worries over his health.

FUTURE WORK

From the studies cited, both those in the literature and those carried out at the Seraphimer Hospital, it appears that psychological and social factors do play an important role in the lives of subjects who ultimately develop myocardial infarction. How these psychological factors interact with known genetic and other physical determinants of MI is a compelling question.[34] Is it that psychological reactions to life events greatly influence physiologic risk factors for MI? What are the relationships between personality and smoking, personality and hypertension, or personality and serum lipids?[1, 6, 10, 39, 43]

Interrelationships between psychological, social and physical risk factors for coronary heart disease are currently being investigated in studies of identical twins in Stockholm. As genetic factors are "controlled" in identical twin pairs, differences in CHD between identical twins appear to be related to differences in personalities and life experiences.[22]

Presently, a large questionnaire study is being carried out with 548 subjects belonging to a nation-wide (Sweden) cooperative chain. All subjects are between thirty-five and sixty-four years of age. Response rate to the questionnaire was 93 percent. Individuals in this sample who recently experienced an MI (1970 or 1971) were compared to healthy subjects in terms of which life changes they had recently experienced. Life changes reported by MI survivors were for the year *prior to* their MI. Control subjects answered for a recent year (1970) chosen because it was the modal year of the MI subjects' recent infarctions. A comparison between the MI and control subjects' reported life events is presented in Table V-III.

TABLE V-III. FREQUENCIES OF LIFE CHANGE EVENTS FOR
MI PATIENTS AND CONTROLS*

	Number of Subjects Responding "Yes"	
Life Change Events	*Patients*	*Controls*
Change to a different line of work	2	1
Important change in working hours (overtime work not counted)	6	1
Increased responsibility at work	5	2
Decreased responsibility at work	0	1
Problems with superiors at work	7	1
Threat of being fired	2	1
Wife seriously ill	5	4
Close relative died	3	2
Close friend died	2	1
Change of residence	2	2
Accidents causing absence from work for 3 weeks or more	5	0
Total no. of cases	65	65

*Patients below sixty-five years of age belonging to the nationwide cooperative chain who had developed MI's during 1970 and 1971. Controls individually matched by age, sex and mode of employment, but otherwise randomly selected from the same population.

Finally, a prospective study of nearly 7,000 men working in a large trade union of building construction workers in Stockholm, ages thirty-five to sixty-four years, is in progress. The Schedule of Recent Experience questionnaire is used along with other psychological, social and physical predictor variables. This investigation will be carried out on healthy men followed prospectively over a two-year period. If psychosocial predictors for MI prove to be of significance, this trade union is interested in their use for possible primary prevention experimentation.

REFERENCES

1. Ander, S.: Personality and smoking. Presented at the seminar, Ten Days of Cardiovascular Epidemiology, at Billingehus, 1971.

2. ————, Andersson, F., Lindstrom, B., Sanne, H., and Tibblin, G.: Psykosociala faktorer vid hjärtinfarkt. *Lärkartidningen, 68*: 3965, 1971.

3. Antonowsky, A.: Social class and the major cardiovascular diseases. *J Chronic Dis, 21*:65, 1968.

4. Arlow, J.A.: Identification mechanisms in coronary occlusion. *Psychosom Med,* 7:195, 1945.

5. Bonami, M., and Rime, B.: Approche exploratoire de la personnalite precoronarienne par analyse standardisee de donnees projectives thematiques. *J Psychosom Res, 16*:103-113, 1972.

6. Brod, J., Fencl, V., Hejl, Z., and Zirka, J.: Circulatory changes underlying blood pressure elevation during acute emotional stress (mental arithmetic in normotensive and hypertensive subjects). *Clin Sci, 17*: 259, 1959.

7. Bruhn, J.G., Chandler, B., Miller, M.C., Wolf, S., and Lynn, T.N.: Social aspects of coronary heart disease in two adjacent, ethnically different communities. *Am J Public Health, 56*:1493, 1960.

8. Buell, P., and Breslow, L.: Mortality from coronary heart disease in California men who work long hours. *J Chronic Dis, 11*:615-626, 1960.

9. Cleveland, S.E., and Johnson, D.C.: Personality patterns in young adults with coronary disease. *Psychosom Med, 24*:600, 1962.

10. Carlson, L.A., Levi, L., and Orö, L.: Plasma lipids and urinary excretion of catecholamines in man during experimentally induced emotional stress and their modification by nicotine acid. *J Clin Invest, 47*:1795, 1968.

11. Dunbar, H.F.: *Psychosomatic Diagnosis.* New York, Hoeber, 1943.

12. Forssman, O., and Lindegård, B.: The post-coronary patient; a multidisciplinary investigation of middle-aged Swedish males. *J Psychosom Res, 3*:89, 1958.

13. Friedman, M., and Rosenman, R.H.: Association of specific overt behavior pattern with increases in blood cholesterol, blood clotting time, incidence of arcus senilis and coronary artery disease. *JAMA, 169*:1286, 1959.

14. Gertler, M.M., and White, P.D.: *Coronary Heart Disease in Young Adults.* Cambridge, Harvard University Press, 1954.

15. Gordon, T.: Further mortality experience among Japanese-Americans. *Public Health Report (Wash), 82*:973, 1967.

16. Hinkle, L.E., Jr.: An estimate of the effects of "stress" on the incidence of coronary heart disease in a large industrial population in the United States. Presented at the Oslo symposium on thrombosis, 1971.

17. ————, Whitney, H.L., Lehman, E.W., Dunn, J., Benjamin, B., King, P., Plankun, A., and Flehinger, B.: Occupation, education and coronary heart disease. *Science, 161*:238, 1968.

18. Hrubec, Z., and Zukel, W.J.: Socioeconomic differentials in prognosis following episodes of coronary heart disease. *J Chronic Dis, 23*:881-889, 1971.

19. Kasenen, A., Kallio, V., and Forsstrom, J.: The significance of psychic

and socio-economic stress and other modes of life in the etiology of myocardial infarction. *Ann Med Intern Fenn, 52*: Suppl. 43, 1963.

20. Keys, A. (Ed.): Coronary heart disease in seven countries. *Circulation, 41-42*: Suppl. 1, 1970.

21. Lew, E.A.: Some implications of mortality statistics relating to coronary artery disease. *J Chronic Dis, 6*:192-209, 1957.

22. Liljefors, I., and Rahe, R.H.: An identical twin study of psychosocial factors in coronary heart disease in Sweden. *Psychosom Med, 32*: 523-543, 1970.

23. Lind, E., and Theorell, T.: Sociological characteristics and myocardial infarctions. *J Psychosom Res, 17*:59-73, 1973.

24. Medalie, J.H.: Factors associated with the first myocardial infarction; 5 years' observation of 10,000 adult males. Presented at the symposium on epidemiology and prevention of coronary heart disease, Helsinki, 1972. (Chairman: M. Karvonen)

25. Paffenberger, R.S., Wolf, P.A., Notkin, J., and Thorne, M.C.: Chronic disease in former college students. I. Early precursors of fatal coronary heart disease. *Am J Epidemiol, 83*:314, 1966.

26. Parkes, C.M., Benjamin, B., and Fitzgerald, R.G.: Broken heart: A statistical study of increased mortality among widowers. *Br Med J, 1*: 740, 1969.

27. Rahe, R.H., and Lind, E.: Psycholosocial factors and sudden cardiac death: A pilot study. *J Psychosom Res, 15*:19, 1971.

28. ————, and Paasikivi, J.: Psychosocial factors and myocardial infarction II. An outpatient study in Sweden. *J Psychosom Res, 15*:33, 1971.

29. Rosenman, R.H.: Assessing the risk associated with behavior patterns. *J Med Assn Georgia, 60*:31, 1971.

30. ————, Friedman, M., Jenkins, C.D., Straus, R., Wurm, M., and Kositchek, R.: Clinical studies: Recurring and fatal myocardial infarction in the western collaborative group study. *Am J Cardiol, 19*: 771-775, 1967.

31. Ruskin, H.D., Stein, L.L., Shelsky, J.M., and Bailey, M.A.: MMPI: Comparison between patients with coronary heart disease and their spouses together with other demographic data—a preliminary report. *Scand J Rehab Med, 203*:99-104, 1970.

32. Russek, H.I., and Zohman, B.L.: Relative significance of heredity, diet and occupational stress in coronary heart disease of young adults; based on an analysis of 100 patients between the ages of 25 and 40 years and a similar group of 100 normal control subjects. *Am J Med Sci, 235*:266, 1958.

33. Shekelle, R.B., Ostfeld, A.M., and Paul, O.: Social status and incidence of coronary heart disease. *J Chronic Dis, 22*:381, 1969.

34. Siltanen, P.: Psychological profile of men with coronary heart disease.

Presented at the symposium on epidemiology and prevention of coronary heart disease. Helsinki, 1972. (Chairman: M. Karvonen.)

35. Syme, S.L., Hyman, M.M., and Enterline, P.E.: Some social and cultural factors associated with the occurrence of coronary heart disease. *J Chronic Dis*, 17:277, 1964.

36. Theorell, T., and Rahe, R.H.: Psychosocial factors and myocardial infarction. I. An inpatient study in Sweden. *J Psychosom Res*, 15:25, 1971.

37. ————, and Rahe, R.H.: Behavior and life satisfactions characteristics of Swedish subjects with myocardial infarction. *J Chronic Dis*, 25: 139-147, 1972.

38. Toor, M.A., Katschalsky, A., Agmon, J., and Allalouf, D.: Arteriosclerosis and related factors in immigrants in Israel. *Circulation*, 22:265, 1960.

39. Torgersen, S., and Kringlen, E.: Blood pressure and personality. A study of the relationship between intrapair differences in systolic blood pressure and personality in monozygotic twins. *J Psychosom Res*, 15:183-191, 1971.

40. Valk, J.M. van der, and Groen, J.J.: Personality structure and conflict situation in patients with myocardial infarction. *J Psychosom Res*, 11:41-46, 1967.

41. Weiss, E., Dlin, B., Rollin, H.R., and Bepler, C.R.: Emotional factors in coronary occlusion. *Arch Intern Med*, 99:628, 1957.

42. Wolf, S.: Psychosocial forces in myocardial infarction and sudden death. *Circulation*, 4, Suppl. 4:74-83, 1969.

43. ————, and Goodell, H.: *Harold G. Wolff's Stress and Disease*, 2nd ed. Springfield, Ill., Thomas, 1968.

44. Yater, W.M.: Coronary artery disease in men 18-39 years of age. *Am Heart J*, 36:334-372, 481-526, 683-722, 1948.

Chapter VI

RECENT LIFE CHANGES AND THE ONSET OF MYOCARDIAL INFARCTION AND CORONARY DEATH IN HELSINKI*

RICHARD H. RAHE AND MATTI ROMO

INTRODUCTION

F INLAND has the dubious honor of being among the leading countries in the world for incidence and prevalence rates for coronary heart disease (CHD).[17] In 1969, The Finnish Heart Association began an Ischemic Heart Disease Register and successful attempts have been made to register nearly all subjects who develop acute episodes of CHD in the Helsinki area. Acute episodes of CHD generally result in subjects' hospitalization, especially when due to either myocardial infarction (MI) or severe angina pectoris. Almost two thirds of coronary deaths, however, occur outside of the hospital, generally because of their extremely rapid course.[2,16] Coronary death subjects listed in the Helsinki Ischemic Heart Disease Register comprised all reported cases which occurred both in and outside Helsinki hospitals.

More than two decades of epidemiologic research, in both the United States and in Europe, have resulted in the identification of a number of "risk factors" for subjects prone to develop CHD.[3,4] Serum cholesterol, blood pressure, degree of body fat, signs of glucose intolerance, and cigarette smoking are now well established

*This work was carried out under the direction of Doctor Pentti Siltanen, Head, Research Department of the Finnish Heart Association, and at the Cardiovascular Laboratory, First Department of Medicine, University Central Hospital, Helsinki, Finland.

risk factors. In addition, selected psychosocial characteristics of individuals have also been shown to be of value in identifying persons at high risk to develop CHD.[1,5,12] For example, intense dedication to work, substantial overtime work, a high degree of competitiveness, a tendency to rush against time deadlines, and selected life dissatisfactions have been shown to be important factors. Both these "physical" and "psychosocial" risk factors for CHD, however, focus on subjects' underlying predispositions for the development of this disease. With the possible exception of cigarette smoking, these physical and psychosocial risk factors are not considered to be precipitants of CHD crises—such as MI or sudden death.[14]

Subjects' recent life changes appear to be possible precipitants of numerous disease entities—including crises of CHD.[6-8,15] This report illustrates how subjects' recent life changes, one measurable dimension of their recent life stress, may be quantitatively assessed and useful in a retrospective study of MI and coronary death. This method's promise for prospective studies is presented in the Discussion.

METHODS AND MATERIAL

Criteria for the diagnosis of acute ischemic heart disease are those that have been outlined by a subcommittee of the World Health Organization and are common to all ischemic heart disease registers used throughout several capitals in Europe.[18] Measurements of subjects' recent life changes were carried out by nurse-interviewers utilizing a Finnish translation of the Schedule of Recent Experience (SRE) questionnaire. This questionnaire, described in detail in a previous chapter by Rahe, is composed of forty-two life change event questions. Respondents indicate which, if any, of the life changes they have recently experienced, and if so, in which three-month interval these events occurred over the past two years.

As in previous studies with the SRE, the life change events themselves were scaled to afford life change unit (LCU) weights for the individual life event items. These LCU weights indicate the relative degrees of life change and readjustment required for each life event as perceived by the average individual. Even though previous studies of individuals living in various countries have indicated a high degree of agreement as to these LCU weights, and especially as to the rank ordering of these life change events by LCU values, a rescaling of the forty-two life change events was carried out in Finland on a separate sample of 149 subjects.[7,10] The results of the Finnish scaling study are shown in Table VI-I. Finns who took part in the LCU scaling experiment were healthy men and women covering a wide age range and were not the same individuals gathered from the Ischemic Heart Disease Register.

TABLE VI-I. LIFE CHANGE EVENTS AND THEIR
FINNISH LCU WEIGHTS

Life Change Events	Finnish LCU Weights
I. *Health*	
1. Recent illness (in bed a week or hospitalization)	62
2. Change in heavy physical work, or exercise	19
3. Change in sleeping habits	15
4. Change in eating habits	11
II. *Work*	
5. Recently out of work	50
6. Recently fired from work	50
7. Retirement from farming, forestry or industry	40
8. Change to new type of work	36
9. Change in work responsibilities	29
10. Troubles with boss	22
11. Work or life gone well (awards, achievements, etc.)	20
12. Correspondence courses (home study)	17
13. Change in hours worked a day	13
III. *Home and Family*	
14. Concern over health of family member	54
15. Recently married	50
16. Separation from wife due to marital problems	48
17. Gain of new family member (in the home)	39
18. Separation from wife due to work	34
19. Engaged to be married	32
20. New home improvements	26
21. Son or daughter leaving home	23
22. Wife begun or end work	23
23. Troubles with in-laws	22
24. Change in get-togethers with friends	21
25. Change to a new residence	15
26. Chance in get-togethers with relatives	13
27. Vacation	11
IV. *Personal and Social*	
28. Death of wife	105
29. Divorce	80
30. Held in jail	64
31. Sexual difficulties	41
32. Change in number of arguments with wife	40
33. Death of a close relative	39
34. Financial difficulties	38

35. Major decisions regarding the future	38
36. Death of a close friend	34
37. Unpaid bills leading to threatened legal action	26
38. Recent purchases more than 8000 Fmk ($2000)	22
39. Change in religious or political convictions	20
40. Change in personal habits	12
41. Recent purchases less than 8000 Fmk	11
42. Minor violations of the law	7

Two hundred ninety-two nearly consecutive subjects in the Helsinki Ischemic Heart Disease Register who survived a definitive MI, and were less than sixty-five years of age, were selected to be given the SRE questionnaire. Complete information was collected on 279, or 95 percent, of all possible subjects. The remaining 5 percent of subjects were either too ill to cooperate or refused cooperation. Over approximately the same time period, 286 subjects, less than sixty-five years of age, dying abruptly from CHD were gathered from the Register. Generally the spouses, but on occasion a close relative, of these subjects were contacted for interview with the SRE questionnaire. Twenty-five of the 286 subjects proved to have no spouse and no close relatives from whom life changes information could be obtained. An additional 24 subjects did have such a relative, but the interviewers were unable to make contact with them. Only 11 relatives contacted refused the interview. Hence, complete life change data were collected on 226 coronary death subjects, or 79 percent of all possible cases; in only 5 percent of the cases where relatives were contacted did they refuse to be interviewed.

From results of previous similar investigations, it was hypothesized that subjects developing an MI or suffering coronary death would reveal increasing LCU totals over the two years prior to infarction or death.[6, 9, 11, 15] Because of this hypothesis, plus the fact that comparisons were made between the same groups of individuals over two years' time, the one-tailed t-test for correlated means was used. For intergroup comparisons, however, the standard two-tailed t-test was utilized.

RESULTS

Recent Life Changes and Myocardial Infarction

The 279 survivors of a definitive MI were divided into two subgroups on the basis of their physical health over the two years prior to their infarctions. One hundred thirteen subjects recorded a significant illness, generally of cardiovascular origin, over the two years prior to their infarctions. One hundred sixty-six subjects recalled no illnesses over the two years prior to their infarctions under study. This division of subjects on the basis of their recent health was necessary because it had been previously demonstrated that individuals' life changes are elevated for several months before, during and following a major illness.[8] Only in the cases of subjects who had been in good health over the two years prior to their infarctions could an elevation in their recent life changes be clearly unrelated to pre-infarction illness.

Subjects' mean, quarter-year, LCU totals are shown for the two years prior to their infarctions in Figure VI-1. MI survivors with pre-infarction illnesses demonstrated relatively elevated, quarter-year LCU magnitudes across the entire two years prior to infarction compared to MI survivors without pre-infarction illness. Both subgroups demonstrated significant elevations in their mean, quarter-year, LCU magnitudes over the six months immediately prior to infarction compared to the same time interval one year earlier. (In Scandinavian samples, many life changes are determined by the season of the year, for example, vacations, overtime work during winter, and so forth; the most comparable interval to a six-month period, therefore, is the same chronological time interval of the preceding year.)

The mean, final six-month, LCU total for MI survivors with premorbid illnesses (quarter years 1 and 2) was 74 LCU. The mean, six-month, LCU total for this group of subjects during the comparable interval one year earlier (quarter years 5 and 6) was 52 LCU. This 42 percent increase in subjects' final six-month LCU magnitude was significant at the 0.025 level of confidence.

Similarly, MI survivors in good health over the two years prior to their infarctions demonstrated a mean final six-month (quarter years 1 and 2) LCU magnitude of 39 LCU compared to a mean six-month total of 23 LCU for the corresponding interval one year ealier (quarter years 5 and 6). This 69 percent increase in mean final six-month LCU total was significant at the 0.005 level of confidence.

Intergroup comparisons between MI survivors with and without pre-infarction illnesses indicated that the MI survivors with premorbid illness had significantly higher six-month LCU totals for both quarter years 1 and 2 and quarter years 5 and 6 than did their counter-

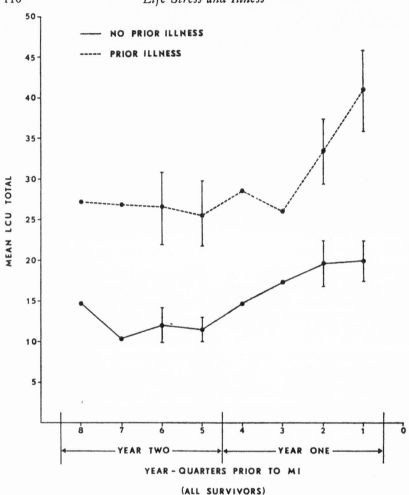

Figure VI-1. Mean, quarter-year, LCU data for MI survivors, with and without pre-infarction illnesses. Standard errors are indicated for quarter years 1, 2, 5 and 6.

parts who reported good health prior to their infarctions (p < 0.01).

Recent Life Changes and Coronary Death

One hundred twenty-six subjects died within an hour from the onset of their symptoms. This subsample was called the "sudden death" group and was itself divisible into 61 subjects who had apparently been healthy prior to their sudden death and 65 subjects who reportedly experienced significant illness over this time period. Similarly, the 100 subjects in the "delayed death" subsample (those who died between one hour and 28 days after onset of symptoms) were divisible into 35 subjects who had apparently suffered no illness during the two-year period prior to death and 49 individuals who reportedly experienced significant illness during this two-year span. In the delayed death group there were 16 remaining subjects diagnosed as having experienced a myocardial infarction prior to death but

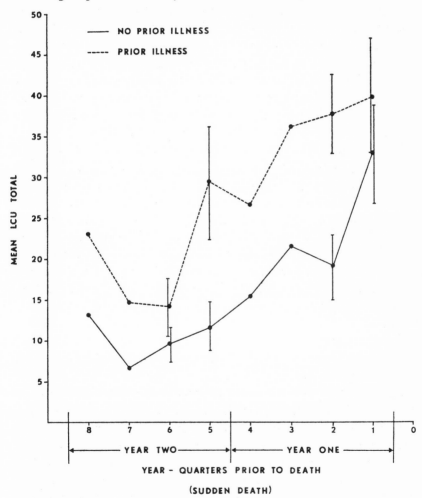

Figure VI-2. Mean, quarter-year, LCU data for sudden death subjects, with and without pre-death illnesses. Standard errors are indicated for quarter years 1, 2, 5 and 6.

where it was possible that they could have died for reasons other than their CHD (such as renal failure). These individuals were excluded from the following life changes analyses.

The eight quarter-year LCU magnitudes registered by the sudden death and delayed death groups over the two years prior to their demise are plotted in Figures VI-2 and VI-3. As both the sudden death and the delayed death groups were subdivided into individuals who were apparently healthy and those who had premorbid illnesses over the final two-year period, each figure had two sets of LCU data. In Figure VI-2 the subsample of sudden death subjects with significant premorbid illness demonstrated relatively elevated quarter-year LCU totals compared to sudden death subjects with no reported pre-death illnesses. Both of these subsamples indicated elevated mean LCU totals for quarter years 1 and 2 in comparison to the corresponding time interval one year earlier, quarter years 5 and 6.

For sudden death subjects who reportedly experienced major illness during the two years prior to their demise, the mean final six-month LCU total (quarter years 1 and 2) was 77 LCU. Their mean six-month LCU total for the latter half of the previous year (quarter years 5 and 6) was 43. This 79 percent increase in the final six-month LCU was statistically significant (p < 0.005). Sudden death subjects with no prior illness had a mean final six-month LCU total of 51 LCU. Compared to the mean six-month LCU total for the final half of the previous years of 21 LCU, this was a 143 percent increase (p < 0.005). Intergroup comparisons between the two subsamples of sudden death subjects indicated that for both quarter years 5 and 6 and 1 and 2, sudden death subjects with prior illness had significantly higher mean six-month LCU totals than did their counterparts with no pre-death illnesses (p < 0.025).

In Figure VI-3 delayed death subjects with previous recent illness showed a relatively elevated mean quarter-year LCU total compared to delayed death subjects without recent illness. Delayed death subjects without prior illness experienced elevated mean final six-month LCU totals (quarter years 1 and 2) compared to the corresponding period (quarter years 5 and 6) one year earlier. Such a final LCU elevation was not seen, however, for delayed death subjects without previous illness.

Delayed death subjects with previous illness over the two years

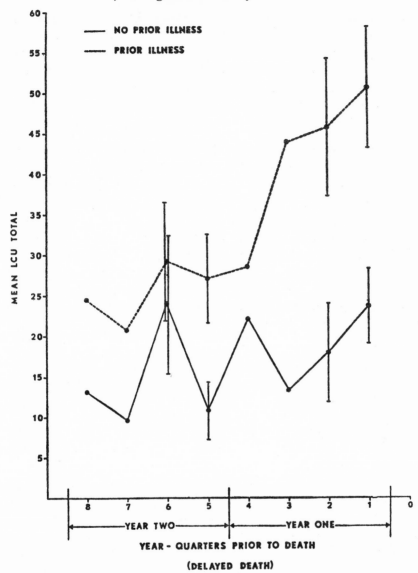

Figure VI-3. Mean, quarter-year, LCU data for delayed death subjects, with and without pre-death illnesses. Standard errors are indicated for quarter years 1, 2, 5 and 6.

prior to death showed a 71 percent LCU increase (from 56 to 96) when quarter years 1 and 2 were compared to quarter years 5 and 6 (p < 0.025). Delayed death subjects with no recent illnesses prior to their demise showed a mean final six-month LCU elevation of only 20 percent (35 versus 42) which was not statistically significant. Intergroup comparisons showed that only in the six-month period immediately prior to death did the delayed death subjects with prior illness demonstrate a significantly higher mean six-month LCU total than subjects who reportedly experienced no pre-death illnesses (p < 0.01).

Distribution of Elevated Recent Life Changes for MI Survivors and Coronary Death Subjects

Not all MI survivors and coronary death subjects showed a final six-month LCU elevation. Some individuals experienced a marked final six-month LCU elevation while others reported no such LCU elevations. In order to examine the distribution of individuals' recent LCU elevations, only MI survivors and coronary death subjects with no premorbid illness over the two years under study were used. In this way, all life changes reported up to the time of infarction or death were presumably due to subjects' accustomed activities of middle age rather than secondary to previous illness.[8]

One hundred sixty-six MI survivors reported no pre-infarction illnesses; 96 coronary death subjects reportedly experienced no illness over the two years prior to their demise. Subjects were divided into the following three categories. (1) This category was comprised of those individuals with a final six-month LCU elevation of at least 100 percent higher than their six-month LCU total for the same time interval one year earlier. In addition, subjects were included in this category if they had registered 0 LCU for quarter years 5 and 6 and a value of 26 LCU or above for quarter years 1 and 2. (A 26 LCU elevation represented the average LCU increase for subjects who reported a final six-month LCU increase of 100 percent.) (2) This category included those subjects with a LCU increase of 1 to 99 percent for the final six-month interval compared to the corresponding time interval one year earlier. In addition, subjects were included in this category if they had registered 0 LCU for quarter years 5 and 6 and then reported 1 to 25 LCU for quarter years 1 and 2. Also included in this category were those few subjects who in quarter years 5 and 6 experienced 26 LCU or more (an "early" LCU elevation), although their final six-month LCU totals were seen to be less than their LCU totals for quarter years 5 and 6. (3) This category was composed of the remaining subjects, those who reportedly experienced 0 to 25 LCU for quarter years 5 and 6 and an equal or lower LCU total for quarter years 1 and 2. In abbreviated terminology: category (1) included subjects with definite or *marked* recent life change elevations; category (2) included those with lesser or *moderate* LCU increases, and category (3) was composed of remaining subjects with neither an early nor late LCU elevation, or *none*. The percentages of MI and coronary death subjects falling into these three categories are shown in Figure VI-4. It can be seen that category (1) subjects (marked elevation) comprised 29 percent of the MI group and 38 percent of the coronary death subjects. Conversely, category (3) subjects comprised 36 percent of MI survivors and 29 percent of coronary death subjects.

The percentages of MI and coronary death subjects falling into these three categories of recent life change elevation varied slightly according to sex, place of birth, and current cigarette smoking habits. If subjects were male and were born in rural Finland, they tended to show higher percentages with marked recent life change elevations than did women or city-born Finns. Subjects who were currently heavy cigarette smokers (more than 1 pack/day) indicated marked recent life change elevations more frequently than subjects who

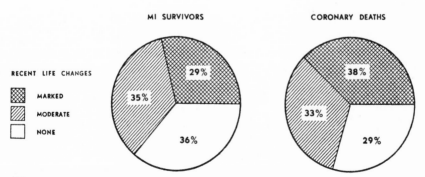

MI(n=166) AND CORONARY DEATH(n=96) SUBJECTS'

DISTRIBUTIONS OF RECENT LIFE CHANGES

MI SURVIVORS   CORONARY DEATHS

RECENT LIFE CHANGES

MARKED   29%   38%
MODERATE 35%   33%
NONE   36%   29%

Figure VI-4. MI and coronary death subjects, without pre-infarction or pre-death illnesses, with marked, moderate and no recent life changes elevations.

smoked less than this amount. These differences were consistently more striking for coronary death subjects than for MI survivors; however, the differences were only statistically significant (p < 0.01) in the case of coronary death heavy smokers (67 percent of whom had marked recent life change elevations) versus coronary death moderate smokers (21 percent had marked elevations). Age, marital status and medical histories of hypertension, diabetes, angina pectoris or intermittent claudication did not show any relationship to the distribution of subjects into the above three categories of recent life change elevation.

DISCUSSION

MI survivors, with and without pre-infarction illness, demonstrated significant increases in their final six-month LCU totals compared to the corresponding time interval one year earlier. This final six-month LCU elevation was seen despite a relatively elevated LCU baseline for those subjects with pre-infarction illnesses. Hence, an increase in LCU magnitudes appeared to herald the onset of new (MI) disease.

With the exception of a relatively small number (n = 35) of delayed death subjects with no reported illness during the two years prior to their demise, significant elevations were also seen in final six-month LCU totals for subjects suffering sudden or delayed death. The two sudden death subsamples and the delayed death subsample with premorbid illness reported between 71 percent and 143 percent elevations in their final six-month LCU totals. Final six-month LCU elevations shown by myocardial infarction subjects ranged between 42 percent and 69 percent. It appeared, then, that subjects with the most severe CHD crises—coronary deaths—generally reported highest recent life change elevations.

The demonstration of significantly increased recent life changes for both MI survivors and coronary death subjects during the final six months prior to infarction or death implies a precipitating influence of these life changes upon the onset of illness or death. It would seem to follow that had not these subjects been exposed to significantly increased life demands, they might not have developed an infarct or coronary death at the time that they did.

A validity study of life changes reported by MI survivors was carried out for 116 of these cases. Spouses were interviewed separately by the nurse-interviewers and answered the recent life change questionnaire in terms of what they knew about their mates' life changes during the past two years. Six-month LCU totals for quarter years 1 and 2 and for quarter years 5 and 6 based upon spouses reports were not found to be significantly different from LCU totals based upon the patients' reports. It seemed, therefore, that spouses' reports could be relied upon to estimate magnitudes of patients' recent life changes. Although it is possible that spouses who have recently been bereaved of their mates will recall life changes differently from spouses whose mates have survived a recent myocardial infarction, it appears impossible to test this hypothesis.

An examination of the percentages of Finnish MI survivors and coronary death subjects who reportedly experienced marked, moderate and no recent life change elevations can be compared to percentages of MI and sudden death subjects who show marked, moderate and no elevations of serum cholesterol or systolic blood pressure (BP). Data for these two well-established "physical" risk factors for CHD have been taken from a large American prospective study of 3,049 middle-aged men followed for the development of CHD over 4½ years.[12] Two hundred of these American men developed a definitive MI; 57 others died from CHD during the follow-up interval. Figure VI-5 shows the distribution of these MI survivors and coronary death subjects for marked, moderate and no serum cholesterol and systolic BP elevations. (Markedly high serum cholesterol values were those above 259 mg%, moderate values were between 220 mg% and 259 mg%, and low values were less than 220 mg%. Similarly, markedly elevated systolic BP values were those greater than 160 mm Hg, moderately high values were betweeen 120 and 159 mm Hg, and low values were less than 120 mm Hg.) Subjects with markedly elevated serum cholesterol levels accounted for 29 percent of MI survivors and 50 percent of coronary death subjects, while those with low levels were 36 percent of MI survivors and 12 percent of coronary death subjects. Subjects with marked elevations in systolic BP were only 13 percent of MI survivors and 15 percent of coronary death subjects, while those with low levels were 18 percent of MI survivors and 12 percent of coronary death subjects.

An enormous challenge for preventive medicine today is to try to identify individuals highly susceptible to development of near-future

Life Stress and Illness

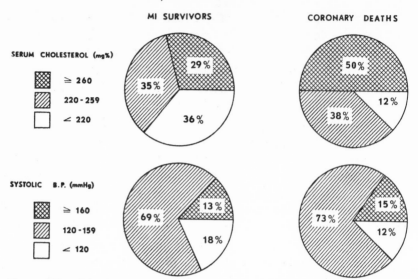

Figure VI-5. MI and coronary death subjects, (American study) distributions for serum cholesterol and systolic blood pressure according to those with marked, moderate and no elevations. (From Rosenman, R.H., et al.: *Am J Cardiol, 19*:773, 1967.)

CHD crises such as myocardial infarction or coronary death. Once again, using data from the American prospective study, of all subjects with systolic blood pressures greater than 160 mm Hg, approximately 5.4 percent developed either MI or coronary death during the following year; of all subjects who had serum cholesterol values greater than 260 mg%, approximately 3.1 percent developed either MI or a coronary death during the following year.[18] Therefore, between 95 and 97 percent of all subjects with either of these high levels of blood pressure or serum cholesterol risk for developing CHD did *not* develop MI or coronary death the following year. Perhaps a major utility of including precipitating factors for CHD in future prospective studies is that factors such as recent life changes may predict higher percentages of subjects prone to develop MI or coronary death during the following year than seems to be the present capacity of subjects' predisposing physical risk factors alone.

Finally, it is currently planned to examine available autopsy data upon the Finnish coronary death subjects as to degrees of coronary atherosclerosis, heart size, previous infarctions, and evidence for recent infarction and/or thrombosis at the time of death. The possibility would then exist to test the hypothesis that coronary death subjects with little evidence of long-standing or severe CHD may be individuals with pronounced recent life change elevations. Because subjects with definite recent life change elevations may have had concomitant high levels of circulating catecholamines as a reaction to their life changes, they may have thereby been more disposed to coronary death secondary to arrhythmias. On the other hand, coronary death subjects with no recent life change elevations may have been those with greater coronary atherosclerosis, greater heart size, and more evidence of chronic degenerative cardiac disease who died primarily from cardiac muscle failure.

REFERENCES

1. Friedman, M., and Rosenman, R.H.: Association of specific overt behavior pattern with blood and cardiovascular findings. *JAMA, 169*:1286-1296, 1959.
2. Gordon, T., and Kannel, W.B.: Premature mortality from CHD: The Framingham study. *JAMA, 215*:1617, 1971.
3. Kannel, W.B., Castelli, W.P., and McNamara, P.M.: The coronary profile; twelve-year follow-up in the Framingham study. *J Occup Med, 9*:611-619, 1967.
4. Keys, A. (Ed.): Coronary heart disease in seven countries. *Circulation* (Supplement), *41*:1-185, 1970.
5. Liljefors, I., and Rahe, R.H.: An identical twin study of psychosocial factors in coronary heart disease in Sweden. *Psychosom Med, 32*: 523-542, 1970.
6. Rahe, R.H.: Life crisis and health change. In May, Philip R.A. and Wittenborn, J.R. (Eds.): *Psychotropic Drug Response: Advances in Prediction.* Springfield, Ill., Thomas, 1969.
7. ————: Multi-cultural correlations of life change scaling: America, Japan, Denmark, and Sweden. *J Psychosom Res, 13*:191-195, 1969.
8. ————, and Arthur, R.J.: Life events surrounding illness onset. *J Psychosom Res, 11*:341-345, 1968.
9. ————, and Lind, E.: Psychosocial factors and sudden cardiac death: A pilot study. *J Psychosom Res, 15*:19-24, 1971.
10. ————, Lundberg, U., Bennett, L., et al.: The social readjustment rating scale: A comparative study of Swedes and Americans. *J Psychosom Res, 15*:241-249, 1971.
11. ————, and Paasikivi, J.: Psychosocial factors and myocardial infarction. II. An outpatient study in Sweden. *J Psychosom Res, 15*:33-39, 1971.
12. Rosenman, R.H., Friedman, M., Jenkins, C.D., et al.: Recurring and

120   *Life Stress and Illness*

fatal myocardial infarction in the western collaborative group study. *Am J Cardiol, 19*:771, 1967.

13. ————, Friedman, M., Straus, R., et al.: Coronary heart disease in the western collaborative group study. *J Chronic Dis, 23*:173-190, 1970.

14. Spain, D.M., and Bradess, V.A.: Sudden death from coronary heart disease. Survival time, frequency of thrombi, and cigarette smoking. *Dis Chest, 58*:107-110, 1970.

15. Theorell, T., and Rahe, R.H.: Psychosocial factors and myocardial infarction. I: An inpatient study in Sweden. *J Psychosom Res, 15*: 25-31, 1971.

16. Wikland, B.: Medically unattended cases of ischemic heart disease in a defined population. *Acta Med Scand,* Suppl. 524, 1971.

17. World Health Organization, Epidemiological and vital statistics report, Vol. 20, No. 1. Geneva, 1967.

18. World Health Organization, Technical report series. Report of a WHO expert committee on Ischemic Heart Disease registers. Copenhagen, 1967.

Chapter VII

LIFE CHANGES IN RANDOM SAMPLES
OF MIDDLE-AGED MEN

SUZANNE ANDER, BODIL LINDSTRÖM AND GÖSTA TIBBLIN

IT HAS BEEN SHOWN by Rahe and others that onset of disease is often preceded by an increased amount of life changes. Our hypothesis is that life changes, like smoking and alcohol consumption, increase wear and tear on the organism. Therefore, it is of interest to measure life changes.

In order to develop an adequate measuring instrument, we conducted a series of studies of random samples, in certain age groups, from the total male population in Göteborg on the west coast of Sweden. A forty-three-item questionnaire was constructed based on an earlier Swedish translation of the SRE questionnaires by Rahe and Theorell. This questionnaire was given to 241 men who were fifty-two years of age, 84 men who were sixty-two years old, and 81 men who were sixty-five years old. They were instructed to report their life changes during the preceding year.

We wanted to know the number of life changes in the different age groups and also how the subjects perceived the intensities of their life changes. Therefore, each event that had occurred was scaled by the subject on a five-step severity scale: (1) a minor change that did not have much effect, (2) a moderate change, (3) a relatively big change, (4) a very big change and (5) a total change of one's entire life situation.

RESULTS

The frequency of life events in the total group studied (men aged

52, 62 and 65 years) is presented in Table VII-I. The distribution of the severity scalings for each life change event is also presented in the table. (The sum of the percentages in the five scale categories is not always 100 percent, because some of the subjects gave a "yes" answer but did not scale the life change.) It is clear from Table VII-I that the life events tend to be graded differently by different subjects.

TABLE VII-I. FREQUENCY OF LIFE CHANGES IN A RANDOM SAMPLE OF SWEDISH MEN AGED FIFTY-TWO TO SIXTY-FIVE

Life Change Events	Percentage Who Answered Each Life Change "Yes"	Percentage of "Yes" Subjects Choosing the Various Severity Scores				
		1	2	3	4	5
Change of income	42.2	36	34	15	3	4
Visit a doctor because of illness	31.2	38	28	16	10	4
Wife being ill	21.8	21	20	26	11	4
Change in financial state	17.9	15	42	22	7	3
Change in working hours	16.9	36	25	16	12	4
Courses because of work	16.2	42	24	20	0	1
Change in health	15.7	17	27	30	8	5
Close relative being severely sick	15.5	19	25	24	11	3
Change in working responsibility	15.2	11	35	26	15	5
Change in personal habits	14.5	10	29	24	15	12
Change in housing conditions	14.0	51	19	11	4	4
Death of close relative	13.5	27	25	18	11	4
Family member leaving home	13.0	42	19	25	6	4
Change in work condition	12.0	33	25	25	6	8
Change in getting together	9.3	29	32	26	5	0
Conflicts with coworkers	8.6	17	49	23	6	6
Change in residence	7.9	22	31	25	6	13
Visit a doctor due to accident	7.6	58	10	10	6	6
Death of a close friend	7.4	20	23	27	0	7
Other specific change in work	7.1	14	17	38	17	10
Separation from wife (work)	7.1	55	21	10	0	0
Wife start or stop work	6.9	39	21	7	0	4
Problems with boss	6.6	19	37	22	15	4
Change to different kind of work	5.9	33	29	8	13	13
Arguments with wife	5.7	43	26	13	13	0
Change in recreation habits	5.7	4	43	30	4	0
Unemployed some part of the year	5.2	19	24	38	0	5
Family problems	4.9	10	60	20	10	0
Threat of being fired from work	3.7	7	27	13	13	40
Retirement from work	3.7	20	0	20	7	13
Other specific changes concerning relatives, friends	3.7	13	33	27	13	0
In-law troubles	3.4	64	14	7	7	0
Starting or leaving a second job	3.2	23	30	30	0	0

Other specific changes in family condition	3.2	15	15	8	15	31
Problems concerning relatives	2.0	25	25	25	25	0
Marriage	1.2	20	0	20	0	0
Marital separation due to argument	0.9	25	25	25	0	25
Birth or adoption of child	0.9	0	25	0	0	0
New person in household	0.7	0	66	0	0	33
Divorce started or finished	0.7	0	0	0	66	33
Death of wife	0.5	0	0	0	0	100
Total Subjects	407					

When working with random samples of the population, it is evident that in the very old age groups the number of men still holding jobs and/or still having wives is less than that found in preretirement men. For example, in our samples the men having jobs, wives and children may report a maximum possible score of 215 LCU, while the men lacking these three attributes can answer only twenty out of the forty-three questions and thus reach a maximum possible score of just 100 LCU. We, indeed, found a fall in mean number of life events reported by our subjects with increasing age. Mean number of life change events reported by men aged 52 was 4.0; the mean number for men aged 62 was 3.8; the mean number reported for men 65 was 3.6.

One way of correcting for age differences in life change reporting would be to calculate a "Standard Life Change Total" (SLCT). A formula is given below:

$$\frac{\text{Total number of life changes reported by the individual} \times 100}{\text{Number of questions applicable to the individual}} = \text{Standard Life Change Total (SLCT)}$$

When we used SLCT instead of raw scores, the above-mentioned difference between age groups disappeared.

In sum, the traditional coronary heart disease (CHD) risk factors only partly predict myocardial infarction, and there is evidence that some of these are nonspecific for CHD. Life change was a variable which turned out to be promising in retrospective CHD studies by Rahe and Theorell. The subject's own grading of his life changes may give a more accurate picture than predetermined scores of a particular event. It may also reflect the subject's perception as well as his way of coping with life change events. The chance of the sub-

ject's exposure to many life changes decreases with advancing age.
One way of correcting for this tendency is to use a Standard Life
Change Total formula, such as the one outlined above.

≥⌇⋀⋀⋀⋀⋀⋀⋀⋀⋀⋀⋀⋀⋀⋁⋁⋁⋁≥

Chapter VIII

LIFE EVENT SCALING FOR
RECENCY OF EXPERIENCE

MARDI J. HOROWITZ, CATHY SCHAEFER AND PAUL COONEY

CONSIDERABLE EFFORT, apparent elsewhere in this volume, has been invested in the development of inventories of life experience for use in quantifying the degree of stress experienced by the average person. The virtue of this method of quantification is that it obtains relatively reliable self-report data. Persons vary or distort reports of events less than they vary or distort reports of the emotional states and subjective experiences which are reactions to such events. Two major problems occur with the use of this method. One concerns the weighting of disparate events to obtain a composite presumptive stress score. The other concerns weighting of individual variations in assimilation and response to events over selected time periods. The problem of individual variation can be partly controlled by using large groups of subjects and presuming that personality differences will neutralize each other. The problem of weighting events is the topic of this study.

For our own use in experimental stress research, we wished to arrive at a presumptive stress score for subjects entering our laboratory. By "presumptive stress" we mean the probable degree of stress the average person might currently be expected to be experiencing, as the consequence of recent life events. Upon review of the various schedules currently available for scoring life events, we found that other investigators focused on recent events, those within one year or six months. Events were scored differently in terms of the amount of stress they incurred, based on data of subjective valuation, but the exact occurrence of the events was not considered in the weighting process. We became interested in devising a similar instrument with an important difference: events would be weighted according to time of occurrence.

This interest in time-keyed scoring rests on the clinical observation that events have an enduring impact. A person may still not have assimilated or accommodated to events that happened years previously. These past events and more recent ones may, theoretically, pile up an accumulated general loading for psychological stress as Selye has suggested for seemingly disparate physical stressors.[4] We believe that persons could differentially valuate the stress from events according to their recency or remoteness in time, just as subjects had differentially valuated the stress itself from a variety of events.[1-3] An initial study was therefore designed with the following predictions.

PREDICTIONS

1. For any given event, recency will confer higher stress ratings.
2. Events rated as extremely stressful, in contrast with less stressful events, will have slower rates of decline in level of assigned stress weighting over time.
3. Experienced events will be rated more stressful than imagined events at increasingly distant time intervals.
4. Women will rate a standard list of life events as more stressful than men.
5. Older subjects will rate events as more stressful than younger subjects.

The rationale for the first hypothesis is based on everyday and clinical observations: reaction to events are often phasic compositions of (a) intrusive and repetitive ideation, emotion and behavioral responses, and (b) denial, numbing and apathy. Both aspects of general stress response syndromes diminish with time. Nonetheless, severe psychological traumas exert a prolonged effect whereas less major disruptions of life can be assimilated with restoration of the pre-event state of psychological affairs, hence, the second hypothesis of a slower rate of decline in the valuation of events rated as major stressors.

The remaining three hypotheses are less important but are also based on clinical observations. Persons may imagine an event to be quite stressful on impact, but may underestimate the degree to which the effects linger on. As indicated in the third hypothesis, persons who have actually experienced an event may better know the extensiveness of its effects, and therefore would rate distant events as more currently stressful than subjects who have not experienced those events. This hypothesis does not apply to recent events because imagined or anticipated events often appear even more threatening than actual occurrences, an effect which leads to an opposite prediction.

In spite of the fact that women have not been noted to differ from men in their assignment of values for impact of life events, women do seem to more readily admit to emotional responses to life changes; hence, a nonreplication of previous findings is predicted in the fourth hypothesis.[1, 3] Similarly, we predicted that older persons would in general be more experienced and perhaps use less denial. These effects might override the greater openness to admitting emotion in today's younger generation and contribute to higher stress ratings, as stated in the final hypothesis.

METHODS

Our schedule of life events was based on lists used by previous investigators. Efforts were made to have only a single page of items, since there would be several time periods for the valuation of each item. In the interest of clarity, wordings were changed. The resulting format had thirty-four items vertically, and five time spans horizontally (1 week after the event, 1 month, 6 months, 1 year and 3 years after the event). Subjects were asked to place a value in each time box for each item. Two forms were used, varying only in item order. No significant differences were found between forms.

Subjects

Subjects consisted of two main groups of unpaid volunteers. A younger group were college students; an older group were medical center personnel and volunteers. Uncompleted, jocular or illegible protocols were discarded after preliminary scanning (about 15% of the total). The resulting data was from 119 persons, of whom 24 were over thirty years of age, 95 were under thirty, 53 were male, and 66 were female, with the sexes evenly distributed over both age groups.

Procedure

Subjects in groups, as they naturally occur in scheduled lectures, were asked to fill out the forms. To even out sex distribution, a few additional forms were completed individually. Written instructions at the top of the forms described the thirty-four items as life changes which, though they might be either positive or negative experiences, could cause "stress." The following points were made. "Different persons experience stress in different ways. Some people have emotional reactions, others have thought responses, increased numbness, mechanical behavior or physical sensations. What is important here is the global concept of the initial impact and the continuing impact of an event upon a person."

Subjects were asked to imagine how much "stress" they would be under at this moment if a given event had occurred and ended at each of the different time spans—1 week ago, 1 month ago, and so forth. The greatest degree of "stress" they could imagine experiencing was to be rated 100, the most tranquil or least stressful effects were to be rated 0 or very low numbers. They were to choose appropriate numbers between 1 and 100 for each time scale for each item. First, however, they were to go through the list and check those items which they had actually experienced, rate those experienced events in each time zone, and then finally they were to imagine the events they had not experienced, and rate those too.

RESULTS

Recency Versus Remoteness of the Events

The hypothesis that, in terms of current impact, recent events would be rated as more stressful than remote events, was strongly supported by the data. In other words, our subjects concurred with the experimental hypothesis that stressful effects of an event decrease over time because their valuation responses were based on expectations rather than on direct observation of responses to stress. There was unanimity in this judgment: virtually every subject for every event rated the degree of stress as greater if the event had taken place one week ago than if it had taken place one month ago, six months ago, one year ago or three years ago. The means for each event are shown in Table VIII-I.

Rate of Decline in Current Stress with Remoteness of Event

Each event was graphed over time using the means for all subjects, for inexperienced versus experienced subjects, for men versus women, and for older versus younger subjects. To make these graphs, events

TABLE VIII-I. EVENTS RANK ORDERED BY MEAN VALUES
FOR THE FIVE TIME INTERVALS

Events	Mean Scores by Time Interval				
	1 wk	*1 mo*	*6 mo*	*1 yr*	*3 yr*
Death of your child or spouse	92	84	70	53	37
Death of parent, brother or sister	90	78	60	41	28
Jail sentence	84	69	55	42	30
Involved directly in unwanted pregnancy	78	64	50	32	19
Drafted	71	61	48	39	23
Spouse unfaithful without your consent	78	63	46	31	22
Marital separation due to argument	79	66	47	30	17
Divorce or break-up with lover	81	67	45	28	16
Death of a close friend	81	63	45	30	17
Marital separation not due to argument	71	57	42	29	18
Began extra-marital affair	66	56	42	30	22
Miscarriage or stillbirth	77	60	38	23	15
Marriage or reconciliation	63	48	35	23	16
Hospitalization of family member for serious illness	75	52	29	16	9
Broken engagement	70	51	31	17	9
Increased arguments with person you live with	63	44	30	20	14
Major personal physical illness	71	52	26	13	6
Birth of child or adoption	58	43	30	21	17
Lawsuit	65	47	28	16	8
Fired	67	46	27	15	9
Separated from close friend or relative	58	44	28	19	13
Court appearance for serious violation	72	42	25	14	7
Major financial difficulties	66	45	27	14	8
Academic failure (important exam or course)	66	41	21	10	6
Unemployed for one month (if employed regularly)	60	42	21	12	7
Took on a large loan	49	35	25	17	14
Move to another city	51	34	22	12	6
Big change in work or school	54	33	17	10	5
Loss of personally valuable object	53	31	16	10	6
Moderate financial difficulties	47	31	18	11	5
Arguments with supervisor or coworkers	53	25	10	5	3
Minor legal violation	38	19	9	4	2
Took a very important exam	51	14	5	3	2
Move in the same city	28	15	8	4	2

were grouped into sets according to both empirical and logical orders. Five empirical sets, as shown by heavy lines in Table VIII-I, were established according to the magnitudes of intensity given by subjects. Seven logical sets were established by the following categorization:

1. Major deaths (three items)
2. Important separations (five items)

3. Arguments with important persons (three items)
4. Major threats to self or self-image (five items)
5. Moderate to minor threats to self or self-image (six items)
6. Threats to material well-being (five items)
7. General change without negative connotations (seven items)

All graphs showed similar declining slopes with one possible, and not statistically significant, exception: the set of most stressful events tended to a slower rate of decline. This trend is divergent from what one would expect of random statistics in terms of regression to a mean. An illustration of such slopes is presented in Figure VIII-1, which shows the slope for means of the most and least stressful sets of events for women who had experienced the involved events.

Experience Versus Nonexperience of Events

Correlations for the five time intervals on the item set ranked as most stressful indicated that the values placed at the "one week ago"

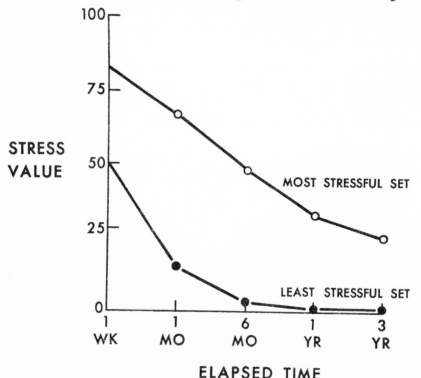

ELAPSED TIME

Figure VIII-1. Slope of decline of scores for the most and least stressful life events, rated by females who had personally experienced these events.

and the "three years ago" interval were predictive of values given for all other time intervals. These time intervals correlated, for all items, with a coefficient of 0.80. Data from these two time intervals were therefore used in analyses of variance (ANOVA). On "threats to material well-being" and "moderate threats to self," the inexperienced group scored higher magnitudes than the experienced group ($F = 4.5$ and 6.6; $p < 0.05$). Experienced persons rated "important separations" as more stressful than did inexperienced persons ($F = 6.8$, $p < 0.05$). Contrary to our hypothesis, no significant differences were found between the experienced and inexperienced group at the three years after the event point of valuation. As might be expected, unexperienced items were valuated with larger deviations on either side of the mean than were experienced items. This suggests a tendency to both exaggerate and deny the effects of anticipated or imagined threats.

TABLE VIII-II. INTERCORRELATIONS AMONG STRESS VALUES FOR FIVE TIME INTERVALS FOR THE ITEM SET "MAJOR DEATHS"*

	1 week ago	1 month ago	6 months ago	1 year ago	3 years ago
1 week ago	1.000	0.800	0.648	0.543	0.300
1 month ago		1.000	0.871	0.756	0.545
6 months ago			1.000	0.920	0.691
1 year ago				1.000	0.816
3 years ago					1.000

*All values are significant ($p < 0.01$); $N = 119$.

Women Versus Men

As predicted, women rated all logical sets as more stressful than did men at the one-week level of remoteness in time (F ratios varied from 8.7 to 28.1; $p < .01$). At the three-year level of remoteness of time from the event, these sex differences disappeared in all categories except for "major threats to self;" women continued to rate these events as significantly more stressful.

Over Thirty Versus under Thirty Years of Age

Contrary to our prediction, the younger group (96 persons) rated events as more stressful than did the older group (24 persons). On the ANOVA, all logical groupings except "arguments" showed significant differences at the one-week point (F ratios varied from 4.5 to 15.5; $p < 0.05$). As observed with sex differences, these subgroup contrasts disappeared by the three-year point of valuation.

Interactions

Three-way analysis of variance between sex, age and experience or not, were computed for the one-week and three-year points of valuation. Of twenty-eight possible interactions at the one-week point, two were significant ($F = 4.6$ and 4.7, $p < 0.05$): sex-age interaction for both "deaths" and "separations" categories. That is, young women rated these categories as significantly more stressful than they did the other categories. At the three-year point, of twenty-eight possibilities, two were significant ($F=4.1$ and 4.7, $p<0.05$): age and experience for "changes with negative evaluation" and the three-way interaction for "major threats to self." That is, young, inexperienced subjects projected threats of "change" as more stressful; young, female, inexperienced subjects rated "major threats to self" as more enduringly stressful.

Comparison with Other Scales

On our thirty-four-item scale, there were sufficient numbered events with wording identical or very similar to those items used by others to allow a comparison of weightings given by our various subject groups.[3] The twenty-four most similar items were rank ordered for each study using the mean weighting by subjects on a 1 to 20 scale of Paykel et al., and the mean on our subjects' weighting using the 1 to 100 scale. The two rank orders correlated significantly with a coefficient of 0.64, a similar coefficient to that for the correlation between the Paykel findings and those of Holmes and Rahe.[1]

There was agreement between ours and the Paykel groups as to the three most stressful events: "death of a child or spouse," "death of a parent, brother, or sister" and "jail sentence." The three items about which there was the most disagreement were "death of a close friend," "marital separation not due to argument" and "marriage and reconciliation." In our sample, all of these were rated as much more stressful than they were in the Paykel sample. It is interesting to note that the Paykel sample rated those items concerned with financial considerations as more stressful than did our subjects. The four items which his subjects ranked as much more stressful were "fired," "major financial difficulties," "unemployed one month" and "loss of a personally valued object." These differences may reflect demographic differences of our younger San Francisco Bay subjects and his older, New Haven area residents.

REFERENCES
1. Holmes, T.H., and Rahe, R.H.: The social readjustment rating scale. *J Psychosom Res, 11*:213-218, 1967.
2. Masuda, M., and Holmes, T.H.: The social readjustment rating scale: A cross-cultural study of Japanese and Americans. *J Psychosom Res, 11*:227-237, 1967.
3. Paykel, E.S., Prusoff, B.A., and Uhlenhuth, E.H.: Scaling of life events. *Arch Gen Psychiatr, 25*:340-347, 1971.
4. Selye, H.: *The Stress of Life.* New York, McGraw-Hill, 1956.

Chapter IX

RECENT LIFE EVENTS AND CLINICAL DEPRESSION*

INTRODUCTION

THE NATURE of the relationship between recent life events and clinical depression has been the subject of as much debate and often bitter controversy as any issue in psychiatry. A number of valid arguments have been advanced against the proposition that most depressions are simple reactions to life events. One is the concept of endogenous depression, based on the clinical observation that some depressions appear to occur in the absence of any preceding stress. In the last decade, multivariate statistical techniques have been applied to this problem.[13] A second, related area concerns biological mechanisms, such as the currently promising catecholamine hypothesis.[25] Here, however, psychological etiology is not precluded since all psychological events must be presumed to have substrates and consequences in brain function so that psychologically and biologically caused depression might well be mediated through a final common neuropharmacological pathway. A third source of dissent concerns those depressions which are preceded by events. Various authors have been sceptical of the role of the stress in these episodes,

*Studies reported in this paper were carried out at Yale University and were supported in part by P.H.S. Grant M.H. 13738 from the National Institute of Mental Health, U.S. Department of Health, Education and Welfare. Collaborative investigators included Gerald L. Klerman, M.D., Jerome Myers, Ph.D., Brigitte A. Prusoff, M.P.H., and E. H. Uhlenhuth, M.D. The author is grateful to Mrs. Myrna Weissman for comments on the manuscript.

134

pointing out that the events may also be consequences of the depression or trivial coincidental occurrences which do not cause depression in most people, and arguing that the true causes of these depressions are to be found in constitutional factors or endogenous mechanisms.[30]

This paper will summarize a series of studies on the relationship between recent life events and clinical depression. The work was carried out at Yale University in collaboration with a number of colleagues, between 1967 and 1971. Some studies in the sequence are still being completed. The general aim of these studies was to apply a more rigorous methodology, particularly use of controls and quantification, to some of the unsettled issues.

METHODOLOGICAL ISSUES

Before these studies are reported it must be acknowledged that it has not, in the past, been easily susceptible to investigation by sophisticated methodology. I have reviewed the difficulties elsewhere.[17] Many apply generally, whatever the context in which stress is studied. They are, however, aggravated by features more specific to depression.

For one thing, truly experimental manipulation of stressful events is impossible and as investigators we must depend on naturally occurring events. However, events do not occur in a vacuum and all of us to some extent bring about the events from which we suffer. In particular, the depressed patient may experience new events as a result of his depression. For instance, he leaves his work because he cannot function in it. His spouse may misunderstand or be unable to tolerate his increased dependency, leading to increased marital friction. To eliminate such consequences of depression we might confine our study to events which clearly preceded the onset of the depression. This onset may be gradual, however, and events following the onset may contribute substantially in a cumulative fashion to the final state.

Another problem arises from the fact that most studies are not prospective. Some investigators have used the model of bereavement for prospective studies.[3,15] However, most bereavements are not followed by depression requiring treatment, and this model may not be entirely appropriate. For the most part studies of clinical depression have therefore been dependent on the patient's reports of events which occurred some time in the past. Inaccuracies of recall for past events may be of major magnitude for anyone. For the depressed patient there may be additional distortions resulting from his current depression which both induce him to seek a cause in the past, and to distort his view of the world by his lowered self-esteem, guilt, hopelessness and helplessness to the point where he may overemphasize the significance of events which did occur.

The need for controls in these studies is obvious. However, it is not always easy to find a suitable group and to hold constant all the relevant factors. In fact, controlled studies have been surprisingly infrequent and only reported in the last decade. Forrest et al.[5] and Hudgens et al.[8] found only weak differences between depressives and medical inpatient controls. However, these may be a biased control group, because there is evidence that life events also cluster prior to medical illness and hospital admission.[24] In a smaller study of recent separations, these were found more common in depressives[26] than in other psychiatric patients. Our own study[20] was the first to use general population controls. Since then Brown et al.[1] have given a preliminary report of a large and careful study employing a similar control group.

A further serious problem, at least until recently, has been the absence of any effective methodology to measure stress in quantitative terms. Precipitation in depression is rarely all or none, frequently partial. This kind of situation requires a quantitative measure to do it justice. Until the last few years no attempts had been made to apply quantitative methods to life stress. The recent pioneering work of Holmes and Rahe[7] has opened exciting new possibilities in this regard.

These are some of the methodological problems to which we have been obliged to seek solutions in carrying out our studies. Overcoming them does in fact present a good deal of difficulty and it is doubtful if any single study can guard against all of them.

COMPARISONS BETWEEN DEPRESSIVES AND GENERAL POPULATION CONTROLS

Data collection in our controlled study took place in 1967.[20] The depressed subjects were 185 depressed patients studied in collaboration with Gerald Klerman. A representative variety of treatment facilities in New Haven, Connecticut, were screened and all patients satisfying research criteria for depression studied further. About half were outpatients, the remainder being treated in inpatient units and day hospitals.

The control subjects were derived from a concurrent general population epidemiological survey of a mental health catchment area of New Haven containing a representative sample of the city's population.[14] In this study a total of 938 households were systematically sampled and one adult was selected at random from each for interview. From this large sample, a sub-sample of 185 subjects was obtained, each matched with an individual of the depressed patient sample for sex, age (in decades), marital status, race and social class.

Information regarding life events was obtained at interview. The depressed patients received an initial psychiatric evaluation. To avoid distortions due to depression, this initial interview did not cover life events. Some weeks after the initial evaluation, when the patients' symptoms were much improved, they were seen by a research assistant interviewer. She administered a semistructured interview covering life events. The control subjects were interviewed by research assistant interviewers in their homes. The interview for life events came near the end of a probing two-hour interview concerning psychiatric symptoms and social role function.

Information collected covered the occurrence of sixty-one events, including most relevant areas of life experiences. These were modified for analysis to thirty-three by condensation of some of the categories, and the omission of some events where there was a possibility of reporting differences between the two groups. The time period for which events were recorded was six months. For the depressed patients, the period was that immediately prior to the onset of the current depressive episode which had been defined in symptomatic terms at the previous interview. This time period was chosen to exclude events which might reflect consequences rather than causes of depression. The median length of illness was four months. For the controls the period was slightly different in timing, being the six months immediately prior to the interview.

We set out to ask two questions of these data: (1) Are life events more frequent just prior to the onset of the depressive episode among patients than in a comparable period in the control sample?

and (2) if so, are all life events more frequent, or only certain types? The first comparison made was of total number of reported events. The findings were striking. Overall, the depressed patients reported three times as many events as their matched controls. The depressed patients reported a mean of 1.69 events per patient in the six-month period. The controls reported a mean of 0.59 per subject.

Frequencies of the individual events were next compared, as shown in Table IX-I. For each event, the significance of difference between the two groups was tested, using x^2 with Yates' correction where appropriate. The increased frequency of total events was paralleled by increased frequency of most of the individual events. For eight events the differences reached statistical significance. These events were increase in arguments with spouse, marital separation, changing to a new type of work which here included starting work for the first time or after a long absence, death of immediate family member, serious illness of family member, departure of family member from home, serious personal physical illness, and substantial change in work conditions. Most of the other events were also reported more frequently in the depressives, but they occurred too infrequently in either group for differences to achieve statistical significance.

EVENT CATEGORIES

This leads to the second research question: Do all events, or only certain types of events, distinguish depressed patients from controls? The question is one of generality versus specificity of stress. Here we turn to an important issue, that of the meaning of the event, or the connotations within it which render it liable to induce depression. The literature on depression has laid emphasis on certain types of events, notably losses of various sorts. On the other hand, a much more general approach has tended to apply in the psychosomatic literature, and was adopted for instance by Holmes and Rahe[7] in their scaling of life events, which they applied profitably to the occurrence of somatic illness. Their scaling depended solely on the magnitude of life change necessitated by life events irrespective of more specific aspects. Does this kind of model also apply to the genesis of depression? In order to examine this issue, events were grouped into categories according to several alternative, but partly overlapping, sets of criteria. For each category frequencies were cal-

TABLE IX-I. FREQUENCIES OF LIFE EVENTS BY DEPRESSIVES AND POPULATION CONTROLS*

Events	Depressed Patients	Controls	Significance†
1. Increase in arguments with spouse	39	1	< .01
2. Marital separation	23	2	< .01
3. Start new type of work	17	1	< .01
4. Change in work conditions	27	11	< .05
5. Serious personal illness	21	7	< .05
6. Death in immediate family member	16	4	< .05
7. Serious illness of family member	23	9	< .05
8. Family member leaves home	6	0	< .05
9. Move	36	25	ns
10. New person in home	11	6	ns
11. Major financial problems	8	3	ns
12. Pregnancy	7	4	ns
13. Unemployed	7	5	ns
14. Court appearance	6	2	ns
15. Childbirth	6	2	ns
16. Lawsuit	6	3	ns
17. Engagement	0	4	ns
18. Demotion	3	0	ns
19. Change schools	3	0	ns
20. Child engaged	4	3	ns
21. Promotion	3	4	ns
22. Fired	3	1	ns
23. Leave school	1	3	ns
24. Marriage	3	2	ns
25. Child married	3	2	ns
26. Jail	2	0	ns
27. Son drafted	2	1	ns
28. Birth of child (for father)	1	2	ns
29. Divorce	1	0	ns
30. Business failure	1	1	ns
31. Stillbirth	1	1	ns
32. Pregnancy of wife	0	0	ns
33. Retirement	0	0	ns
Number of cases	185	185	

*Modified from Paykel, E.S., Myers, J.K., Dienelt, M.N., Klerman, G.L., Lindenthal, J.A., and Pepper, M.P.: Life events and depression: a controlled study. *Arch Gen Psychiatr, 21:753, 1969.*
†x^2 (with Yates' correction).

culated in terms of numbers of individuals reporting at least one event from that category.

The first grouping of events was according to the area of life endeavor they involved. Five categories were so derived: employment, health, family, marital and legal. Twenty-five of the thirty-four events could be assigned to one of these. When frequencies were examined the results were somewhat similar in all categories. In each at least twice as many events were reported by depressives as controls. This categorization did not differentiate events.

Another way of looking at events was in terms of a value dimension, based upon cultural norms and social desirability. In terms of general shared values, some events are regarded as undesirable and other events as desirable. In our event list, only a few clearly desirable events had been included, principally such events as promotion, engagement, marriage. A much larger group of events was clearly undesirable, such as demotion, being fired, death of a close family member, major financial problems. This view of events contrasts for instance with the Holmes-Rahe scaling which depended solely on the magnitude of life change, with desirability specifically excluded from consideration, and in which paired events, such as demotion and promotion, involving equal life change in terms of work responsibilities were regarded as equivalent. Experience suggests that undesirable events such as demotion are more likely than desirable equivalents such as promotion to precipitate depression, although the latter may not always be blame-free.

The results shown in Table IX-II tentatively support this view. Undesirable events were reported in both groups of subjects more frequently than desirable events, but this may merely reflect the item content of our list. When depressives were compared with controls, undesirable events were reported much more frequently by the depressives. By contrast, there were no significant differences between the two groups regarding desirable events. Indeed, although not significant, the pattern was reversed, with controls reporting more events than depressives. Here we have a fairly clear indication of differential effects—only certain types of events appear to precede depression.

A third and more specific categorization referred to ten events which involved changes in the immediate social field of the subject. Two classes of events were defined. Entrances referred to those events which involved the introduction of a new person into the social field and exits those events which clearly involved a departure from the social field. The findings are set out in Table IX-III. Exits

TABLE IX-II. INCIDENCE OF DESIRABLE AND UNDESIRABLE EVENTS*

Event Category	Depressed Patients	Controls	Significance†	Events Included In Category
Desirable	6‡	10	ns	Engagement Marriage Promotion
Undesirable	82	31	< .01	Death of family member Separation Demotion Serious illness of family member Jail Major financial problems Unemployment Court appearance Son drafted Divorce Business failure Fired Stillbirth

*Modified from Paykel et al., 1969.[20]
†x^2 (with Yates' correction).
‡Number of individuals reporting at least one event in category.

were much more frequently reported by depressives than controls. Entrances, although reported with almost equal frequency overall, were equally distributed between the two groups. Exits from the social field, of course, correspond closely to a familiar psychiatric concept in relation to depression, that of loss. To reinforce this relationship, in the larger general population sample from whom the controls were drawn, exits were also much more likely than entrances to be associated with minor psychiatric symptoms.[14]

One additional categorization was of interest. The original life events list contained several additional items which referred to arguments or difficulties in interpersonal relations. These were omitted from the final list of events on which the two groups of subjects were compared, because it was felt that the patient group might report these more readily as a result of their recent experience of psychiatric treatment. We did, however, examine them separately, and the findings are shown in Table IX-IV. The differences between

TABLE IX-III. ENTRANCES AND EXITS FROM SOCIAL FIELD*

Event Category	Depressed Patients	Controls	Significance†	Events Included In Category
Entrance	21‡	12	ns	Engagement Marriage Birth of child New person in home
Exit	46	9	< .01	Death of close family member Separation Divorce Family member leaves home Child married Son drafted

*Modified from Paykel et al., 1969.[20]
†x^2 (with Yates' correction).
‡Number of individuals reporting at least one event in category.

patients and controls were striking—ninety patients reported at least one event from this category as opposed to five controls. Although these findings may be at least in part interview artifacts, it seems unlikely that the entire difference is due to reporting errors. This may be another class of event particularly related to the depressive episode.

The patients and controls, although matched, spanned a wide range of sociodemographic characteristics. In order to explore the universality of the findings, the comparisons between depressives and controls on the four most important categories—exits and entrances, undesirable and desirable events—were re-examined in sub-

TABLE IX-IV. INTERPERSONAL DIFFICULTIES OMITTED
FROM MAIN LIST

Depressed Patients	Controls	Significance	Events Included in Category
90*	6	< .01	Arguments with resident family member
			Arguments with nonresident family member or friend
			Arguments with fiance or steady date
			Cease steady dating

*Number of individuals reporting at least one event.

samples broken down by sociodemographic variables. These included three separate age groups (20 to 29, 30 to 44, 45 to 65); males and females; married, formerly married and single; Negroes and Caucasians; and social classes—Classes I, II and III combined, Class IV and Class V. In all these separate groups depressed patients reported significantly more events overall than controls. The same excess was also apparent in exits and undesirable events (except in single patients, where N's were very low). In no sociodemographic group were there significant differences between patients and controls for entrances or desirable events. The main findings, therefore, seem to hold for a wide variety of sociodemographic groups.

SPECIFICITY

Overall these findings strongly support the role of life events in the onset of clinical depression. Moreover, they suggest some degree of specificity in that exits and undesirable events appear particularly related to depression, while their opposites, entrances and desirable events, were not implicated.

How specific is this relationship? At best it can only be considered partial. A highly specific hypothesis would propose that there are certain classes of events which produce depression, and only depression. The evidence does not indicate such a degree of specificity. The excess among depressives included almost every event in our list, except entrances and desirable events. Many subjects reported a cluster of events which, on detailed scrutiny of narrative summaries, suggested a cumulative model of stress. The findings for the exit-entrance and undesirable-desirable categories were important because they were distinctions which discriminated contrasting events and hinted at some kind of specificity. Nevertheless, the range of events reported in excess by the depressives in our study was quite diverse. It would be hard to include all these events under any single formulation, even the commonly suggested one of loss.

Adequate investigation of the degree of specificity also requires attention to the other side of the equation—the disturbances produced. We cannot say from the use of general population controls whether exits from the social field might not equally precede a variety of other psychiatric, or even medical, illnesses. Additional studies are at present under way on two further patient groups, suicide attempters and first admission schizophrenics. However, the events already found to precede depression indicate that a variety of different kinds of events which are in some way noxious, but which do not include all events, converge in preceding depression. Among these, exits and undesirable events are of particular, but not unique, importance.

FOLLOW-UP STUDY

The previous findings used general population controls. Another kind of control, which does not appear to have been exploited in published reports, is the within-patient control provided by follow-up study. This would enable us to deal with the criticism that, whatever the precaution, experiences of psychiatric treatment may render the subject more willing than a nonpsychiatric control to recall and report unpleasant events. It also deals with a different and potentially valid criticism—the possibility that events reported at onset by depressives are primarily reflections of personality disturbance and habitually unstable life patterns and might be reported just as frequently at any other time.

Such a follow-up is not without its own methodological flaws. In our comparison with general population controls, we chose a time period prior to onset for which to record events, so as to avoid those which were consequences rather than causes of depression. For a follow-up, at least in the short term, it is not easy to do this. Many events, occurring soon after recovery, such as return to work and job changes, may be consequences of the recovery itself. However, at least in this situation the biases would inflate figures for the control group, and work in favor of the null hypothesis.

Subsequent to the main data collection, we did carry out a short-term nine-month follow-up study on the depressives.[18] Life event data, which were collected on a randomly selected seventy of the subjects, has not previously been reported. The life event interview technique was basically the same as for the previous interview, with the additional element that the month of occurrence of each event was also recorded. In order to obtain a comparable time period to that for onset, analyses for events were confined to the last six months of the follow-up period. Extensive information regarding symptomatic course and outcome was also collected, and to minimize effects of persistent illness this information was used to select those subjects, thirty in all, who had recovered within three months and remained well for the subsequent six months. The numbers in this crucial follow-up sample were, therefore, somewhat low.

Table IX-V shows the proportion of these subjects reporting the main categories of events, and includes for comparison the figures for patients when ill and for the controls. These are based on the full samples, but findings for the small group of thirty were essentially the same. Frequencies of entrances and desirable events remained low and showed no convincing change. Those for exits and undesirable events fell considerably to about half the frequency at onset, from 25 percent to 10 percent for exits, 45 percent to 23 percent for undesirable events. They still remained a little higher than control values—10 percent versus 5 percent for exits, 23 percent versus 16 percent for undesirable events. In some other respects, the changes appeared to involve patterns of events more than the total number of events. Some events, particularly those related to employment, increased in frequency. On close scrutiny many of these were changes consequent upon the recent illness and recovery. It would require a longer follow-up to establish a clear period of freedom from illness and its effects, and any findings from this small study are clearly only tentative.

Within these limits, this follow-up study does confirm the relationship between depression and the major classes of exits and undesirable events. The failure of these event groups to fall in frequency all the way to control levels probably reflects a mixture of illness residue, reporting bias and the element in event occurrence which is due to habitual maladaptive patterns tending to produce such events.

MAGNITUDE OF EFFECT

Although the differences we found in event occurrence between depressives at onset and normal controls appear relatively large, they

TABLE IX-V. COMPARISON OF ONSET AND RECOVERY GROUPS

	Depressives (Onset)	Depressives (Recovered)	Normal Controls
Entrances	12*	16	10
Desirable events	3	3	5
Exits	25	10	5
Undesirable events	45	23	16
Number of Cases	185	30	185

*Percentages of subjects reporting at least one event from each category.

have to be viewed in their full context. It has often been pointed out that close scrutiny of the events reported by depressives suggests that they can only at best be partial causes. Most of the events reported by the patients in our study and also in other studies were in the range of everyday experience rather than catastrophic. It seems probable that in most cases these events are negotiated without clinical depression. Some other factors must contribute to the development of depression. It is particularly easy to lose sight of the importance of base rates for the population. When the prevalence of a disease state is relatively low, single events will be of limited value in explaining it if they occur with moderate frequency in the general population.[29]

A simple calculation which I have reported previously will illustrate this problem.[17] The difference between depressives and controls for frequencies of exits from the social field in our own study were as large as any reported. We found exits among 46/185 depressives, i.e. 25 percent, and 9/185 controls, i.e. 5 percent. Suppose we accept these figures as accurate. Clearly exits only preceded depression in a minority, albeit substantial, of cases. Let us, however, try to refer these figures to the general population. Accurate figures for the occurrence of clinical depression in the general population are not available.[27] Suppose we take a generous estimate of 2 percent for the incidence of new cases in the six months for which data were collected. If we apply these figures to 10,000 general population subjects we obtain the results given in Table IX-VI. In this group, 200 subjects would become depressed; 50 of these depressions would be preceded by exits. Only 50 of a total of 540 exits (9.2%) would be followed by clinical depression. The large majority of the subjects who experience exits do not become clinically depressed. The greater part of the variance in determining depression must be attributed to something else.

If these incidence estimates were reliable rather than hypothetical, they would comprise suitable data to which to apply epidemiological concepts of attributable and relative risk.[12] The risk of depression in this example among subjects who did not experience exits would be 1.6 percent (150 in 9,460). Subtracting this from 9.2 percent, we obtain an illness rate of 7.6 percent attributable to exits. This is very far from one to one. However, the relative risk

TABLE IX-VI. CALCULATION OF PROPORTION OF EXITS
FOLLOWED BY DEPRESSION

Among 185 depressives:	46 exits in six months = 25%
Among 185 normal controls:	9 exits in six months = 5%
Assuming 2% of the population develop depression in six months,	
then among 10,000 subjects:	9,800 normals, 200 depressives
Among normals:	9,800 x .05 = 490 exits
Among depressives:	200 x .25 = 50 exits
Total exits =	540

Exits followed by depression = $\dfrac{50}{540}$ = 9.2%

is 5.7 (9.2 divided by 1.6) percent. Any effect which increased the incidence of depression six-fold would have to be regarded seriously.

Another way of looking at this issue has been presented by Brown et al.[1] They have devised a concept which they call the "brought-forward" time, corresponding to the amount of time by which the events may be considered on the average to have advanced expectation of a spontaneous onset. Applying the formula to our figures for exits they obtained a brought-forward time of 2.7 years, quite close to the figure of two years for events of markedly threatening implications which they obtained in a similar study of their own. I have also applied their formula to our findings for the occurrence of at least one event of any kind from the list of thirty-three, and obtained a figure of 1.9 years. There appears to be some consistency to these calculations. Although interpretation of the brought-forward time is not entirely straight-forward, the findings to date point to an effect of reasonable, although far from overwhelming, importance.

The calculation in Table IX-VI was of course based on a number of questionable assumptions. The relationship would appear closer if we took a higher incidence for depression so that in effect more subjects experiencing exits became depressed. Something substantial would still remain. It falls under the general rubric of vulnerability or predisposition.

This vulnerability may be seen as having a variety of components, psychological and biological, genetic and environmental. Certain personality types may well be vulnerable to certain classes of events; for instance, clinical experience suggests obsessive personalities are particularly susceptible to events which involve marked changes of routine. Some personalities might be more vulnerable to stressful events of any kind. Previous experience of an event and successful or unsuccessful coping may modify subsequent reactions. Equally vulnerability must also include biological, neuropharmacological elements such as enzyme defects, cyclical changes in function, and variations in metabolic pools of transmitter substances. Genetic elements are clearly important. There may be a host of noxious or protective modifying elements in the current environment, including the detailed circumstances of the stressful event itself, cumulative stress from other recent events, and support from key interpersonal figures. It might be expected that all these would converge in the genesis of the clinical state, the ultimate convergence being in the neurophysiological mechanisms controlling mood.

Future research into the relationship of life events to depression will have to pay much more attention to these crucial interactions with modifying factors. There have been relatively few such systematic studies. It would appear necessary to measure simultaneously stress and the various aspects of vulnerability. Prospective studies of reactions to events, and in the community rather than the psychiatric clinic, will be necessary in the long run before the amount of variance in causation of depression which is due to events can be determined reliably.

SCALING OF LIFE EVENTS

One problem in the studies of depression in the literature is the absence of quantification for life stress. The method of quantification described by Holmes and Rahe[7] opens up new possibilities in this regard. We have used the scores which they described to weight events occurring to our subjects, and have reported some of the findings.[21] However, this procedure was approximate and involved some guesswork, since our event list was not identical with theirs. We therefore undertook, in collaboration with Dr. E. H. Uhlenhuth, a rescaling of the events in our list.[22]

Subjects for this study were a new sample of 373, 213 of them mixed psychiatric patients (predominantly outpatients), 160 relatives of psychiatric patients. The sixty-one life events of our full life events list were set out in a scaling questionnaire. Two forms, with different randomized orders of events, were used alternately. Subjects were asked to make the judgments on a 0 to 20 equal interval rating scale, reproduced on the form. Instructions read as follows:

Below is a list of events that often happen to people. We would like you to think about each event and decide how upsetting it is. Use your own experience and what you know about other people to make your decision. A particular event might be more upsetting to some people than to others. Try to think how upsetting the event would be to the average person.

Below is a list of numbers to show how upsetting the event is. In the blank next to each event, write the number that shows how upsetting that event is. For instance, if you decide it is a little upsetting, write a low number; if it is very upsetting, write a high number. Please be sure to give an answer for every event. Remember, for each event, think about how upsetting it is for all people, the average person, not just you.

The general findings of this study were similar to those obtained by Holmes and Rahe, using a rather different scaling technique. The scaling proved readily feasible. Table IX-VII sets out means and standard deviations of the rating scores, ranked in descending order of magnitude. The mean scores covered almost the complete available range of the scale from 19.33 for death of a child to 2.94 for having a child marry with approval. At the head of the list were events which might be expected to be of major proportions—death of a child, of spouse, being sent to jail, serious financial problems, being fired, miscarriage and stillbirth, and the like. At the lower end of the scale were events which could not be expected to cause much upset.

The low-scoring events appeared to be of two kinds. Some, although they involved moderate life change and readjustment, were desirable in quality. These included marriage of a child with the respondent's approval, becoming pregnant when wanting a baby, engagement, child's engagement, birth or adoption of child, marital reconciliation, promotion and marriage. Some other events in the lower range appeared to be relatively trivial, implying little in the way of either life change or undesirability. Examples included a move within the same city, minor somatic illness and minor legal violation.

One of the advantages of this interval scaling over the ratio scaling used by Holmes and Rahe is that distributions are sufficiently normal for standard deviations to be useful estimates of variability. As

TABLE IX-VII. MEAN SCORES FOR PERCEPTIONS OF LIFE EVENTS*

Rank Order	Event	Mean	S.D.
1	Death of child	19.33	2.22
2	Death of spouse	18.76	3.21
3	Jail sentence	17.60	3.56
4	Death of family member	17.21	3.69
5	Spouse unfaithful	16.78	4.14
6	Major financial difficulties	16.57	3.83
7	Business failure	16.46	3.71
8	Fired	16.45	4.20
9	Miscarriage or stillbirth	16.34	4.59
10	Divorce	16.18	4.95
11	Marital separation due to argument	15.93	4.55
12	Court appearance	15.79	4.26
13	Unwanted pregnancy	15.57	5.18
14	Major illness of family member	15.30	4.15
15	Unemployed for one month	15.26	4.38
16	Death of close friend	15.18	4.55
17	Demotion	15.05	4.57
18	Major personal illness	14.61	4.44
19	Begin extramarital affair	14.09	5.40
20	Loss of personally valuable object	14.07	4.90
21	Law suit	13.78	5.02
22	Academic failure	13.52	5.07
23	Child married (not approved)	13.24	5.36
24	Break engagement	13.23	5.31
25	Increased arguments with spouse	13.02	4.91
26	Increased arguments with family member	12.83	5.15
27	Increased arguments with fiance	12.66	4.96
28	Take a large loan	12.64	5.43
29	Son drafted	12.32	5.75
30	Troubles with boss or coworker	12.21	5.06
31	Argument with nonresident family member	12.11	5.09
32	Move to another country	11.37	6.05
33	Menopause	11.02	5.78
34	Moderate financial difficulties	10.96	4.98
35	Separation from significant person	10.68	5.18
36	Take important exam	10.44	5.08
37	Marital separation not due to argument	10.33	5.68
38	Change in work hours	9.96	5.49
39	New person in household	9.71	5.45
40	Retirement	9.33	6.02
41	Change in work conditions	9.23	5.12
42	Change in line of work	8.84	5.38
43	Cease steady dating	8.80	5.34

*Modified from Paykel, Prusoff, and Uhlenhuth, 1971.[22]
Possible scale values were 0-20; N = 373.

TABLE IX-VII (Continued)

Rank Order	Event	Mean	S.D.
44	Move to another city	8.52	5.59
45	Change in schools	8.15	5.39
46	Cease education	7.65	5.73
47	Child leaves home	7.20	4.96
48	Marital reconciliation	6.95	5.91
49	Minor legal violation	6.05	4.78
50	Birth of live child	5.91	5.70
51	Wife becomes pregnant	5.67	5.23
52	Marriage	5.61	5.67
53	Promotion	5.39	4.90
54	Minor personal illness	5.20	4.29
55	Move in same city	5.14	4.49
56	Birth of child (father) or adoption	5.13	5.45
57	Begin education	5.09	4.48
58	Child becomes engaged	4.53	4.57
59	Become engaged	3.70	4.64
60	Wanted pregnancy	3.56	5.39
61	Child married (approved)	2.94	3.75

shown in Table IX-VII they ranged from highs of 6.05 for emigration and 5.91 for marital reconciliation, to lows of 2.22 for death of child and 3.21 for death of spouse. Most of them lay between 4 and 5.5. When compared with the scale range these standard deviations appeared moderate in magnitude. Estimates would not be much use for single individuals since two standard deviations on either side of the mean spanned a moderate range. For group application they appeared adequate. Confidence limits for the sample means for these 373 subjects were certainly good, the 95 percent limits for most events being about ± 0.5.

Consistency between different sociodemographic groups was examined by correlating mean scaling scores and was found to be very high, confirming the report of Holmes and Rahe.[7] None of the correlations was below .980. We are at present extending this scaling to an English sample at St. George's to explore cross-national consistency.

PERCEPTIONS OF STRESS

The primary purpose of this scaling study was to provide weighting scores for use in other applications. However, the scores also reveal which events are perceived as stressful. They spanned a considerable diversity. Among the events ranking in the top half of the list some were separations, including deaths, divorce and marital separation. Others involved blows to the self-esteem, such as demotion, business failure, being fired, and academic failure. Financial threats were implied in major financial difficulties, taking a large loan and some other events; threats to physical integrity in major somatic illness.

Not surprisingly, these events include many of the events found related to the onset of depression in the controlled study. There was a particularly striking finding when we examined exits and entrances. Among sixty-one events included in this study there were six which were entrances to the social field, and thirteen which were exits. Table IX-VIII gives the mean scaling scores for the events in these two groups. There were marked differences between them. Almost all exits were scaled high and all the entrances low. There was scarcely any overlap; only three exits scored lower than the highest entrances. Only one exit, child marries with respondent's approval, overlapped to any marked degree, and it virtually specified desirability. It would appear then that exits and entrances are perceived as very different in stressful implications by most individuals, and in a way which coincides with their relation to depression. Depending on this viewpoint, these findings can be regarded both as providing validating evidence for the scale, and as supporting the importance of the exit-entrance distinction.

We have also explored some other ways of classifying events. Scores for events generally regarded as undesirable were a good deal higher than those for desirable events, but that was almost implied in the scaling process. We also tried to distinguish those events which were at least partly under the respondent's control and could be initiated by him from those outside his control and found that the uncontrolled events were perceived as more stressful.

Some of these findings may be a function of the scaling concept we used, the degree to which each event was regarded as upsetting, which although not precise, has connotations of distress akin to depression. In using this concept we diverged from Holmes and Rahe who asked their subjects to scale events in terms of the amount of adjustment to life change they necessitated, irrespective of desirability. This view represents an advance over the frequent assumption that desirable change entails negligible stress. Nevertheless, it

TABLE IX-VIII. MEAN SCALING SCORES FOR EXITS AND
ENTRANCES IN THE SOCIAL FIELD*

EXITS:	*Score*
Death of child	19.3
Death of spouse	18.7
Death of family member	17.2
Divorce	16.2
Marital separation due to argument	15.9
Death of close friend	15.2
Child marries (not approved)	13.2
Break engagement	13.2
Separation from significant person	10.7
Marital separation (not due to argument)	10.3
Cease steady dating	8.8
Child leaves home for other reasons	7.2
Child marries (approved)	2.9
ENTRANCES:	
New person in household	9.7
Marital reconciliation	7.0
Birth of child (for mother)	5.9
Marriage	5.6
Birth of child or adoption (father)	5.1
Become engaged.	3.7

*Modified from Paykel and Uhlenhuth, 1972.[23]

seemed to us that implications of events involving distress or un-desirability were important in relation to psychiatric disorder. We therefore selected a concept with connotations of distress, and did not exclude desirability in our instructions or in the naming of our events.

Some evidence from a small additional sample suggests this choice was appropriate, at least regarding the genesis of depression.[23] Forty subjects were involved; all were white female psychiatric patients aged twenty to forty. Twenty scaled the events using the technique of our main study; twenty used differing instructions specifying adjustment to life change, rather than upset, as the concept to be scaled. Seventeen events were scored significantly differently by the two techniques. Table IX-IX shows the findings for the thirteen exits and six entrances. There was a striking distinction between them. All six entrances were scaled significantly lower for upset than adjustment, so that on the upsetting scale they fell in the lower half and mostly near the bottom. Only two of the thirteen exits were scored lower for upset, and once again one of these was the event, child marries with approval, which specified desirability. In other words it appears that the concept of "upsetting" is particularly relevant to the role of events as precipitants of depression. This raises the intriguing possibility that different implications of events may be relevant in different circumstances. For instance, Holmes and Rahe have been particularly interested in psychosomatic disorders. The model of adjustment to life change has been widely used in that context, and may be particularly applicable, even if the distress implied by the concept of upsetting is more appropriate to depression. In the long run this possibility will have to be investigated more thoroughly and directly by documenting the event experience of different patient groups.

ENDOGENOUS DEPRESSIONS

So far this discussion has ignored the possibility of endogenous depressions unrelated to life events. In order to consider this issue,

TABLE IX-IX. EXITS AND ENTRANCES IN THE SOCIAL FIELD:
MEAN SCALING SCORES BY CONCEPTS OF ADJUSTMENT
AND UPSETTING*

Exits:	Adjustment Mean	Upsetting Mean	Significance of Difference
Death of child	19.50	19.70	ns
Death of spouse	18.00	18.35	ns
Death of family member	17.40	19.10	ns
Divorce	16.60	17.75	ns
Marital separation due to argument	15.35	17.10	ns
Death of close friend	13.70	14.85	ns
Child marries (not approved)	13.15	14.85	ns
Break engagement	11.00	13.85	ns
Separation from significant person	9.25	11.25	ns
Marital separation (not due to argument)	11.00	12.95	ns
Cease steady dating	8.10	10.60	ns
Child leaves home for other reasons	10.40	6.70	< .05
Child marries (approved)	8.35	3.65	< .05
Entrances:			
New person in household	14.25	7.75	< .001
Marital reconciliation	14.30	6.85	< .001
Birth of child (for mother)	10.75	3.05	< .001
Marriage	16.30	5.70	< .001
Birth of child or adoption (father)	12.95	5.95	< .001
Become engaged	7.65	3.37	< .05
Number of cases	20	20	

*Modified from Paykel and Uhlenhuth, 1972.[23]

we must return to the 185 depressives who were included in the controlled study.

We attempted to estimate the proportion of depressives in that study whose episodes would be regarded as endogenous. Using the diminished thirty-three-item life events listed employed for the controlled study, 19 percent of depressives reported no events in the six months preceding onset. However, using the full sixty-one-item list, only 7 percent did so. At the same time some of the events reported by those experiencing one or two events were quite trivial and probably unrelated to depression. Indeed, counting the overall number of events does not provide a very useful way of looking at the data since it ignores the kind of event.

One alternative way of estimating the proportion of endogenous depressives was by clinical judgment. Narrative summaries and case histories were used, after the main study had been completed, to make overall judgments as to precipitation, using all the available evidence, including such aspects as time sequences of events and illness, and content of illness. In terms of these about 15 percent of episodes appeared unprecipitated. The majority of depressions appeared to at least involve some element of life stress.

The judgment as to whether a depression is endogenous or reactive, although it features prominently in the literature, is in fact a very difficult one to make. It is uncommon that the answer can be a clear-cut yes or no. More often there are some events, but they are not sufficiently overwhelming to be a sole cause of the depression, and the situation is one of partial and ambiguous precipitation. This is the kind of circumstance which requires a quantitative rather than categorical approach. The main purpose of the scaling study was to provide quantitation. We have elsewhere reported findings using Holmes-Rahe weights for this approach.[21] Here I will report newer findings using weights derived from our own scaling study.

The weights shown in Table IX-VII were applied to the events reported by the depressed patients in the controlled study. As the main tool a summed score, the total stress score, was derived for each patient by adding weights for all the events that he reported. Since the assumption of additivity of events which underlies this has not been proven empirically, an alternative score, the maximal event score, was also derived by taking the single event weight for the highest event reported by the patient. In fact the two scores gave closely similar results.

Figure IX-1 shows a frequency histogram for the total stress score. The majority of these subjects reported total stress much in excess of the score of 10 that would derive from a single event of minor implications in our 0 to 20 scale, or the score of 20 that would indicate a single catastrophe. These high scores were derived from clusters of moderately stressful events. The general shape of the distribution was skewed with a tail in the high scores. It has been argued in the literature that if endogenous and reactive depressions can be clearly separated, the distribution of scores on a measure distinguishing them ought to be bimodal.[2] Usually this has been examined using multivariate scores derived from factor analysis or discriminant function analysis, and predominantly reflecting sympton picture. If we adopted a highly purist view, however, and concerned ourselves solely with precipitant stress, the frequency distribution shown would provide one test of this hypothesis. Clearly this distribution is not bimodal. Thompson and Hendrie[28] recently reported similar findings using Holmes-Rahe scores. The curve also illustrates the difficulty of making the judgment as to whether an episode is actually precipitated. The range of 10 to 30, which in terms of the meaning of the scores for individual events might provide a reasonable cutoff point, coincides with the peak of the distribution, where small changes in cutoff level will make major changes in the subjects classified in each category.

STRESS AND SYMPTOM PATTERN

As usually employed the concept of endogenous depression involves a fusion of the endogenous-reactive and psychotic-neurotic dichotomies. Endogenous depressives are considered to be distinguished not only by absence of precipitant events, but also by certain specific symptom features, such as severe depression with psychomotor retardation, and by premorbid personalities regarded as non-neurotic, obsessional or stable.[9, 11] In recent years a number of studies have used factor analysis to explore this issue, and most have reported a dimension with weights reflecting the contrast between endogenous and neurotic depression.[13]

One problem with all these studies is that the judgment as to the presence or absence of psychological precipitants is usually made in

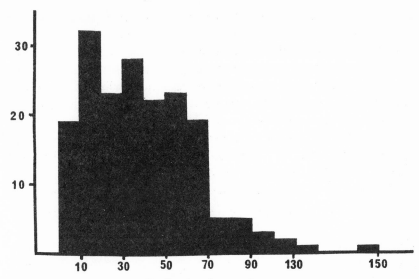

Figure IX-1. Frequency distribution for total stress scores.

the form of a simple yes-no judgment, the serious inadequacies of which have already been discussed. Moreover, this judgment is usually made by the same rater who rates symptoms and personality, so that it is very easy for rater bias to produce a spurious correlation in accordance with the investigator's preconceptions.

In order to avoid these potential biases we employed the quantified measure of precipitant stress which has already been presented, and used separate raters for life stress, symptoms and personality. The life event information was collected after clinical improvement by a research assistant unaware of the detailed sympton pattern. The symptoms were rated by a psychiatrist at initial interview, without any knowledge of life event material. Ratings were made on an expanded and modified version of the Hamilton Depression Scale[6] in which items were on seven-point scales with closely defined anchor points. Personality was rated by self-report after clinical improvement, using the Maudsley Personality Inventory[4] which contains an N scale intended to measure premorbid neuroticism.

In order to explore the degree to which symptoms clustered into patterns, principal component analysis was carried out on the symptom data alone.[19] Twenty-eight symptoms were included. The first three factors accounted respectively for 15.23 percent, 7.81 percent and 6.29 percent of the variance and were interpretable. Factor loadings are set out in Table IX-X. The first factor showed positive loading on almost all items and appeared to be a severity factor. The second factor was bipolar, contrasting negative loadings on a pattern of retardation, morning worsening, and quality of depression different from the usual experience, against positive loadings on irritability, anxiety, reactivity, initial and middle insomnia, self-pity and depersonalization. This closely resembled bipolar factors contrasting endogenous and neurotic depression reported by Kiloh and Garside[10] and Carney et al.[2] The third factor was also bipolar. It appeared to contrast negative loadings on typical depressive symp-

TABLE IX-X. FACTOR ANALYSIS OF CLINICAL RATINGS*

	Factor Loadings		
Rating Items:†	Factor I	Factor II	Factor III
Retardation	.34	—.39	—.17
Distinct quality	.31	—.39	.16
Diurnal variation (worse AM high)	.23	—.30	.26
Agitation	.45	—.22	.00
Insight	.42	—.21	.20
Depressive delusions	.55	—.21	—.01
Guilt	.40	—.19	—.18
Pessimism and hopelessness	.54	—.14	—.41
Hostility	.27	—.09	—.31
Constipation	.55	—.06	—.07
Work and interests	.60	—.02	.12
Change of appetite (anorexia high)	.39	.05	—.07
Helplessness	.57	.08	—.02
Delayed insomnia	.28	.09	.04
Depressed feelings	.46	.12	—.30
Energy and fatigue	.39	.12	.16
Obsessional symptoms	.20	.22	.10
Anxiety—psychic	.32	.22	.58
Hypochondriasis	.49	.22	.39
Paranoid ideas	.08	.28	.03
Suicidal tendencies	.31	.28	—.49
Depersonalization	.37	.30	.13
Self-pity	.33	.32	—.14
Middle insomnia	.16	.37	—.16
Reactivity	—.51	.39	.01
Initial insomnia	.35	.47	—.32
Anxiety—somatic	.26	.49	.61
Irritability	—.11	.55	—.32

*Modified from Paykel, Klerman, and Prusoff, 1970.[19]
†Items listed in order of loadings on Factor II.

toms and hostility with positive loadings on anxiety and hypochondriasis.

The second factor in this analysis provided strong evidence that the symptoms said to be characteristic of endogenous and neurotic depression tended to cluster together so as to form two contrasting patterns. It remained to examine the relationship of this symptomatic distinction to stress and personality. Factor scores for individuals were calculated on the three factors, and were correlated with stress and personality measures.

Table IX-XI shows the correlations between the factors and the two alternative stress scores. The total stress score correlated significantly with factor II in the predicted direction that patients with endogenous symptom pattern reported less life stress, but the correlation was very low, .15, and there was an almost significant correlation with factor III. For the maximal event score the correlation was only with factor III, in a direction that patients with an admixture of anxiety showed less stress than patients with a more typical depressive pattern. Thus, the relationship between stress and symptom pattern, although in the predicted direction, was so weak as to be trivial and was not entirely specific to the endogenous-neurotic symptom dimension. Moreover, increasing age showed a substantial correlation both with the endogenous pole of factor II, and with the total stress score. When this effect was partialled out, the correlation between factor II and the total stress score fell to well below significance.

By contrast for the Maudsley Personality Inventory the only significant correlation was with factor II. It was of reasonable magnitude, .35, and in the predicted direction that patients with neurotic premorbid personality tended to show neurotic rather than endogenous symptoms. The third element which might be expected in

TABLE IX-XI. CORRELATIONS BETWEEN SYMPTOM FACTORS AND
STRESS SCORES (UPSETTING SCALE)

Factor Score	Total Stress Score	Maximal Event Score
I, Severity	—.08	.04
II, Neurotic (+) vs. Endogenous (—)	.15*	.07
III, Anxious (+) vs. Depressed (—)	—.14	—.15*

*p < .05

these relationships, a correlation between stress and neuroticism was entirely absent, the correlations between neuroticism and either stress score being near zero.

Further analysis of these data using cluster analysis techniques for grouping individuals showed evidence of four groups, rather than two. These groups have been described in detail elsewhere.[16] One group was typically psychotic. The other three groups shared some features regarded as characteristic of neurotic depressives, but showed further differences among themselves. One consisted of middle-aged depressives with considerable anxiety, one of depressives showing hostility in addition to depression, and one of younger patients whose depressive episodes developed on a background of personality disorders. Here, too, life stress was only a weak differentiator between groups, and most patients in all groups showed some evidence of preceding and potentially stressful events.

Overall then it would appear that stress is only a weak differentiator in clinical classification. Syndromes corresponding to those in the literature can readily be delineated, predominantly on a symptomatic basis. Premorbid neurotic personality relates moderately strongly to these. When assessed separately, presence or absence of precipitant stress relates only very weakly. Although some depressions appear entirely endogenous, they are a relatively small proportion of the total. More often the judgment of precipitant stress is not a clear-cut one and is better viewed as a quantitative dimension.

CONCLUSIONS

This paper has summarized a series of studies into aspects of the relationship between life events and depression. No attempt has been made to review the relevant literature in any detail, but it should be clear that these studies are merely contributions from one research group to a field that has received wide study. Rigorous clinical research methodology is particularly difficult to apply here, and all studies need replication.

In our studies we have depended on a retrospective collection of life event information, with a number of precautions to cut down contamination from the effects of recent depression. We have used as controls general population subjects and the same patients after recovery. For a third type of control, that of other patient groups, we await completion of current studies. These last controls are important; they may reveal the extent to which the findings are specific to depression, or apply to various diagnoses. We have also attempted to apply quantification based on consensus scaling.

The comparison of depressed patients with general population controls provides strong support for a general relationship between life stress and the onset of clinical depression. Certain kinds of events, notably events regarded as undesirable and exits from the social field appear particularly involved, although the range of events preceding depression is quite diverse, and certainly too wide for any formulation to comprehend them all. Follow-up data showing a considerable drop in frequencies supports the particular importance of these two classes of events at onset.

In terms of event perceptions a considerable range of events is perceived as stressful. Exits appear prominent among these and clearly separated from entrances, although this is only one of a number of similar distinctions. The scaling concept of adjustment to life change distinguishes entrances from exits less than does that of upset.

Although the majority of depressive episodes are preceded by at least some potentially stressful life events, some depressions do occur in the absence of any important overt stress. The clues which they provide on neuropharmacological investigation may have wider generality, but these endogenous depressions appear to represent a small proportion of all clinical depressions. Application of a quantified methology indicates that presence or absence of precipitation is a quantitative dimension rather than a clear-cut separation. Symptom pictures do tend to occur together to produce the patterns described as typical of endogenous or psychotic depression. These patterns, however, show little relationship to presence or absence of precipitant stress; the psychotic-neurotic dichotomy bears only a weak relationship to the endogenous-reactive one. Although most depressions bear some relationship to life events, the proportion of variance in causation which can be attributed to the life event is relatively small. The event falls on some kind of fertile soil, and a host of factors modify the reaction to it. While it is easy to specify these factors in broad terms, their detailed interactions with events have not been adequately studied.

More generally it seems likely that depression is a final common pathway towards which a number of causes, recent and previous, converge. The complexities are such that even in the single case several elements are likely to underlie the development of clinical depression at one point in time. It would appear that it is the interaction between the life event and predisposing factors which is usually of crucial importance. If the focus shifts, as in due course it should, to prevention, these issues will loom large. The events reported by depressives are mostly part of everyday experience, and the inevitable consequences of personal and familial growth, development, and aging. It is difficult to see how such events could ever be eliminated. If life events are to provide approaches for prevention, it would seem that the most likely pathways are those involving modification of the reaction to the event, via these protective or aggravating interacting factors.

REFERENCES

1. Brown, G.W., Harris, T.O., and Peto, S.: Life events and psychiatric disorder: 2. Nature of causal link. *Psychol Med*, in press.
2. Carney, M.W.P., Roth, M., and Garside, R.F.: The diagnosis of depressive syndromes and the prediction of E.C.T. response. *Br J Psychiatr*, *111*:659-674, 1965.
3. Clayton, P., Desmarais, L., and Winokur, G.: A study of normal bereavement. *Am J Psychiatr*, *125*:170, 1968.
4. Eysenck, H.S.: *The Manual of Maudsley Personality Inventory*. London, University of London Press, 1959.
5. Forrest, A.D., Fraser, R.H., and Priest, R.G.: Environmental factors in depressive illness. *Br J Psychiatr*, *111*:243-253, 1965.
6. Hamilton, M.: A rating scale for depression. *J Neurol Neurosurg Psychiatr*, *23*:56-62, 1960.
7. Holmes, T.H., and Rahe, R.H.: The social readjustment rating scale. *J Psychosom Res*, *11*:213-218, 1967.
8. Hudgens, R.W., Morrison, J.R., and Barchha, R.: Life events and onset of primary affective disorders: A study of 40 hospitalized patients and 40 controls. *Arch Gen Psychiatr*, *16*:134-145, 1967.
9. Kendell, R.E.: *The Classification of Depressive Illnesses*. Maudsley Monograph No. 18. London, Oxford University Press, 1968.
10. Kiloh, L.G., and Garside, R.F.: The independence of neurotic depression and endogenous depression. *Br J Psychiatr*, *109*:451-463, 1963.
11. Klerman, G.L.: Clinical research in depression. *Arch Gen Psychiatr*, *24*: 305-319, 1971.
12. MacMahon, B., and Pugh, T.F.: *Epidemiology: Principles and Methods*. Boston, Little Brown and Co., 1970.

13. Mendels, J., and Cochrane, C.: The nosology of depression: The endogenous-reactive concept. *Am J Psychiatr, 124*:1-11, 1968.
14. Myers, J.K., Lindenthal, J.J., and Pepper, M.P.: Life events and psychiatric impairment. *J Nerv Ment Dis, 152*:149-157, 1971.
15. Parkes, C.M.: The first year of bereavement: A longitudinal study of the reaction of London widows to the death of their husbands. *Br J Psychiatr, 33*:444-467, 1970.
16. Paykel, E.S.: Classification of depressed patients: A cluster analysis derived grouping. *Br J Psychiatr, 118*:275-288, 1971.
17. ————: Life events and acute depression. In Scott, J.P., and Senay, E.C. (Eds.): *Separation and Depression: Clinical and Research Aspects.* Amer Assoc Advanc Sci, in press.
18. ————, and Dienelt, M.N.: Suicide attempts following acute depression. *J Nerv Ment Dis, 153*:234-243, 1971.
19. Paykel, E.S., Klerman, G.L., and Prusoff, B.A.: Treatment setting and clinical depression. *Arch Gen Psychiatr 22*:11-21, 1970.
20. ————, Myers, J.K., Dienelt, M.N., Klerman, G.L., Lindenthal, J.J., and Pepper, M.P.: Life events and depression: A controlled study. *Arch Gen Psychiatr, 21*:753-760, 1969.
21. ————, Prusoff, B.A., and Klerman, G.L.: The endogenous-neurotic continuum in depression: Rater independence and factor distributions. *J Psychiatr Res, 8*:73-90, 1971.
22. ————, Prusoff, B.A., and Uhlenhuth, E.H.: Scaling of life events. *Arch Gen Psychiatr, 25*:340-347, 1971.
23. ————, and Uhlenhuth, E.H.: Rating the magnitude of life stress. *Can Psychiatr Assoc J, 17*:93-100, 1972.
24. Rahe, R.H.: Life-change measurement as a predictor of illness. *Proc R Soc Med, 61*:1124-1128, 1968.
25. Schildkraut, J.J., and Kety, S.S.: Biogenic amines and emotion. *Science, 156*:21-30, 1967.
26. Sethi, B.B.: Relationship of separation to depression. *Arch Gen Psychiatr, 10*:486-495, 1964.
27. Silverman, C.: *The Epidemiology of Depression.* Baltimore, Johns Hopkins Press, 1968.
28. Thompson, K.C., and Hendrie, H.C.: Environmental stress in primary depressive illness. *Arch Gen Psychiatr, 26*:130-132, 1972.
29. Wender, P.H.: On necessary and sufficient conditions in psychiatric explanation. *Arch Gen Psychiatr, 16*:41-47, 1967.
30. Winokur, G., Clayton, P.J., and Reich, T.: *Manic Depressive Illness.* St. Louis, Mosby Co., 1969.

≋\/\/\/\/\/\/\/\/\/\/\/\/\/\/\≋

Chapter X

LIFE-EVENTS AND THE ONSET OF DEPRESSIVE AND SCHIZOPHRENIC CONDITIONS*

GEORGE W. BROWN

THE CONCEPT OF DISEASE is having a rough time—not least in psychiatry. Many emphasize the undesirable social and personal consequences of disease labeling and at times go so far as to question the usefulness of the whole notion of disease in psychiatry.[13, 20, 23] Whatever the merits of such views, the day-to-day use of disease concepts in clinical practice should not be confused with the use of diagnostic labels in a research setting as descriptive tools.[25] To reject the act of classification as the basis of a scientific enterprise because of shortcomings of diagnostic labels in a clinical context is unwarranted and short-sighted. Simple methods of classification are a minimal prerequisite for any research undertaking. I have in mind placing individuals together because of common characteristics; schemes that assume some underlying dimension are another matter. The use of diagnostic labels need not imply acceptance of theoretical notions nor any of the etiological or treatment implications commonly held about the diagnostic groups. Nor does it mean that current clinical labels will prove useful, but it seems foolish to ignore them.

*The work on schizophrenia and depression has been supported by the Foundation Fund for Research in Psychiatry, the Medical Research Council and the Social Science Research Council. We should like to thank the many psychiatrists working at hospitals in Southwark whose generous cooperation has made this work possible. Drs. John Copeland and Michael Kelleher assisted in some of the clinical work.

There have been a number of recent interesting suggestions that disease categories may for certain purposes be profitably combined. Syme,[22] for example, has pointed out that although the age-adjusted coronary heart disease rate is very much higher in New York and California than North Dakota and Nebraska, so is the all cause death rate. Coronary heart disease accounts for about 35 percent of all deaths in New York and California, but this proportion persists in almost every state of the country. "The problem, then, is not to explain why New York and California have a higher *coronary* rate than North Dakota and Nebraska, but why New York and California have a higher *death rate* than North Dakota and Nebraska." He goes on to suggest that perhaps research workers ought to be thinking about the forces in the social environment which lead to breakdown of health in general. Recently, Antonovsky[1] has explored this idea and suggested the use of the concept of a breakdown syndrome in stress research in addition to investigating specific diagnostic groups. The work of Rahe and his colleagues[17] is an example of the usefulness of combining all disease groups to form one "outcome variable." Studies of life events in psychiatry have almost all either combined diagnostic categories or dealt only with single diagnostic groups. This is somewhat surprising when one recalls the success of classical studies such as that of Faris and Dunham[11] in Chicago in relating differing living conditions to separate diagnostic groups.

Recent work in London suggests that as far as schizophrenic and depressive conditions are concerned, it is vital to separate diagnostic groups for both practical and theoretical reasons. Not only do quite different types of life events tend to be involved in provoking these conditions, but the kind of causal role that the events play in onset is also radically different. I want first to describe the two London studies and then go on to discuss some of the implications of the work. Details of these studies have been reported previously.[2, 5-7, 9]

THE DEPRESSIVE AND SCHIZOPHRENIC STUDIES

Some characteristics of the main populations used in the two studies are given in Table X-I. The schizophrenic study has been completed; the material for the depressive study has been collected, but the data are still being analyzed.

TABLE X-I. SOME CHARACTERISTICS OF THE MAIN SAMPLES IN THE
SCHIZOPHRENIC AND DEPRESSIVE STUDIES

	Schizophrenic Study		Depressive Study	
	Patients	General Population	Patients	General Population
Number of cases	50	325	114	152*
Sex	Both	Both	Women	Women
Age range	15-65	15-65	18-65	18-65
Mean age	32.7	33.8	42.7	38.5†
Treatment	Inpatient	Nil	Inpatient (41) Outpatient (73)	Nil
Selection	Consecutive admissions, if onset within 3/12	Random, 6 local firms	Consecutive admissions, if onset within one year	Random households and random selection within each from women aged 18-65
Area of residence	Mainly Camberwell	Camberwell	Camberwell	Camberwell
Period covered in interview	3/12 prior to onset	3/12 prior to interview	1 yr prior to admission	1 yr prior to interview
Refusal rate	Nil	5%	1%	14%

*This number is an interim one: in all 220 women in the community have been interviewed, the results of this paper being based on the data available, i.e. on 152 with 26 cases excluded for some purposes. The main calculations have been carried out on the total with essentially similar results.

†Mean age includes the 26 cases.

Depressive Study

1. PATIENT SELECTION. The main group of psychiatric patients were 114 women, 73 inpatients and 41 outpatients, resident in Camberwell, a community of about 175,000 in South London. Only persons aged between 18 and 65 and resident in Camberwell were eligible for inclusion. Records of admissions were screened regularly to identify possible subjects. All had been given a primary diagnosis of depression uncomplicated by any underlying condition, such as alcoholism or organic psychosis. Patients were included if there had been an important change in their condition in the twelve months prior to admission (inpatients) or first outpatient contact (outpatients).

2. INTERVIEW. The patients were interviewed by one of two re-

search workers who had at least several months' experience with the interview schedules and rating scales. For the first fifty patients the other interviewer saw a close relative. The interviewer obtained from the patients information about life events, long-term difficulties and other social data as well as information about onset. The same material was collected from the relative. The total interviewing time with patient and relative took about six hours. All interviews were tape recorded and ratings made later by the interviewer, quite independently of knowledge from the interviewer concerned with the other informant. There were a number of sections to these interviews: (1) clinical information; (2) the events which have occurred are established; (3) characteristics of the event and circumstances surrounding the patient's reaction to it; and (4) long-term difficulties, support from the environment and various miscellaneous measures.

3. COMPARISON GROUP. Two hundred and fifty ratable units were randomly selected from the borough rating registers. Where the unit contained several households, a household was selected at random from these. A list of women in the household was then obtained by a personal visit and a woman then selected at random for interview. Two hundred and twenty women were interviewed.

Interviews were carried out by one of three research workers after several months of training. The interviews with the comparison group were exactly the same as the patient interviews, the year before the day of interview being covered, except that a screening schedule was used to determine current mental state. This instrument was developed by psychiatrists working on the US/UK Diagnostic Project at the Institute of Psychiatry. Two psychiatrists visited a subsample of the women to check on the ratings made of whether the person had been a "psychiatric case" during the previous year. Eighty-four percent agreement was reached. The interviewers had all been trained in the use of the schedule by the two psychiatrists. Women with no more than a mild disturbance of mood were not included in the disturbed group. The following subject, for example, was considered borderline and was not included: in response to standard questions she reported that she had been exhausted and worn out during the day for four weeks before interview; that she had had difficulty in relaxing, was fidgety and restless with some feelings of muscular tension; that she had been depressed intermittently and was less talkative; that although she still went to work, she otherwise found it too much effort to go out. She was irritable with her husband, intolerant over small things, and took things out on her child. She said she had felt like crying occasionally but had cried only once.

Schizophrenic Study

For the schizophrenic series patients were accepted only if onset occurred within the thirteen weeks prior to hospital admission. All patients were examined shortly after admission by a research psychiatrist and the diagnosis judged on conventional Kraepelinian grounds (see Wing et al.[24] for a detailed account of the procedure employed). Fifty cases were studied; for all but five, the hospital diagnosis was one of schizophrenia. A random sample of employees from six local firms were used as a comparison group. There were 115 clerical workers, 60 skilled factory workers, 148 semi-skilled or unskilled factory workers, and 54 building workers.

MEASUREMENT OF LIVE EVENTS

Both studies paid particular attention to various methodological problems involved in the study of life events and the onset of psychiatric disorders.[9] For the present account I will discuss only one of these: the grounds on which life events should be included in the study. Should the investigator include all events reported to have been found distressing or should he apply some external set of criteria to determine inclusion? Classification based on reports of distress may lead to serious bias. Patients and relatives may, in recalling the past, exaggerate the significance of events as a means of coming to terms with the illness. Moreover, even if the patient truly *did* experience the event as he described, this may mean no more than that the event occurred just before the onset of the disorder and the event and its consequences were found distressing because in such circumstances even minor incidents may at times be experienced as upsetting.

Because of such difficulties we have moved away from using the patient's definition of what has been found upsetting and instead apply a common set of criteria of our own. Early in the interview we establish whether certain events have occurred irrespective of how the person felt about them. At this stage we avoid any mention of what has been found distressing or exciting and simply go through an extensive list of events which on common sense grounds are likely to be emotionally important for many people. In order to do this we defined, *before* each study began, both the types of event and the persons to be covered in the questions. Events were asked about which could be potentially dated to a definite point in time and which involved danger, significant changes in health, status or way of life, the promise of these, or important fulfillments. By and large only events occurring to the patient or close relatives (parents, siblings, children and spouse) were covered. On a few occasions particularly dramatic incidents (such as death) concerning more distant kin, or even strangers, were included as long as the subject was present and directly involved.

Detailed notes had to be developed about what should be included as an event which required little judgment on the part of the interviewer. This was done because if this kind of decision had been left to the interviewer's judgment, he might have been influenced by the way the event was reported. It was essential to decide on such details before the main interview began. Once the problem of what was to be included had been settled, a lengthy list of questions was designed to ask about particular events in the degree of detail required.

In this way events were asked about and recalled without the respondent having to report what had or had not been distressing. Incidents which would be expected to be trivial on common sense grounds, but which were in fact highly disturbing for personal reasons, were at times excluded. Events were included only if they conformed to criteria laid down before the interviewing began; as already pointed out, these criteria were based on a judgment that the event would be emotionally important for most people. The method therefore provides, we believe, a minimal estimate of the role of events in the onset and development of psychiatric conditions.

In the depressive study we also pay a good deal of attention, once the basic data about the occurrence of events has been collected, to the characteristics of the events themselves. There is a good deal of general questioning and various rating scales are used to describe each event. They include, for example, preparation for the event (in terms of amount of warning and nature of previous experience) and implications of the event for the person's future (how far it involved change in patterns of interaction or routine and so on). These ratings give each event a more specific or personal meaning than that given by the general descriptive category. The particular circumstances surrounding the illness of a close relative, or a change of house, for example, may differ quite radically according to the seriousness of the illness, the identity of the relative, or whether the house move was sought or enforced as a result of eviction.

The most general of these ratings, *severity of threatening implications*, will be referred to later in this paper. It is a four-point scale ("marked," "moderate," "some," "little or none") and refers to the threat or difficulty implied by the event once the more immediate effects are over. The consequences of many events are fairly completely resolved within a week, such as unexpectedly having to deliver a neighbor's baby. Others, such as discovery of a daughter's thefts, have longer term implications for the future. The interviewer makes a common sense judgment of how unpleasant and threatening the event would be for most people about one week after its occurrence. The rating takes into account all the circumstances—past, present and future—surrounding the event in a particular case, but deliberately ignores the person's own reported reaction to the event. (This information was excluded from the material used for rating.) The reasons for this are the same as those put forward for rejecting the respondent's definition of the event: reported severity may be influenced by "an effort after meaning" to do with the illness, or the event may have been reacted to severely simply because it coincided with the onset of the disorder. Thus events such as desertion by one's husband, or death of a parent, would be rated "marked," irrespective of the person's reported reaction; while a son's engagement to an unexceptional girl would be rated "none," even if his mother said she had found it very distressing and could not bear the thought of him leaving home. A moderate rating would be given to a mother whose son (seen daily) announced he was going to emigrate to Canada. All circumstances surrounding the event are taken into account. In rating a husband's hospital admission, for instance, factors such as still being in an intensive care unit at the end of a week, the doctor saying his condition could be serious, and the fact that he had a previous attack would be considered in the rating.*

*We refer to this measure as the contextual long-term threat rating. Ratings for the scale have reasonably satisfactory interrater reliability when two raters are used

SCHIZOPHRENIC STUDY RESULTS
Schizophrenic patients were studied for the three months before onset. The entire difference appeared to occur in the three-week period immediately before onset: the rate of events was three times greater in this time than that in the general population sample, but outside these three weeks the rate was much the same in the two groups. In the three-week period immediately before onset the rates were 88 and 22 events per 100 persons for the patient and comparison group, respectively. Sixty percent of patients had at least one event in this period compared with 20 percent in the comparison group.[5]

A wide range of life events was apparently involved in provoking onset of acute schizophrenic episodes. All events were classified in terms of a simple descriptive scheme such as "job change," "change of residence" and "health change," and also by whether the subject was the person mainly involved in the event (or equally involved with someone else). Such events are termed subject-focused. If the subject's wife was badly injured in a car accident but the subject himself was little harmed, the event is not subject-focused. If they had been both equally injured, the event is classified as "joint" and will be treated as subject-focused for my present purpose. Patients were much more likely to be the focus of events, 80 percent compared with 53 percent in the general population ($p < .001$, 1 df). Figure X-1 shows that differences between the patient group and general population were particularly large for changes of job, changes of residence and health changes occurring to the subject.

The general population group was not selected to be comparable to the patient group other than by a rough age matching. The two groups were in fact comparable in age, and there were only small differences in other background demographic factors. Age and size of household were the background factors most highly related to the rate of events, although sex and marital status showed statistically significant associations.[5] However, when allowance was made for these factors by standardizing the patient material on the larger general population group the results were hardly affected.

(product-moment correlation of 0.75). However, because it was considered a particularly difficult rating, four investigators, including the interviewer, met weekly during the collection of material to rate events independently, discuss inconsistencies and come to an agreed rating.

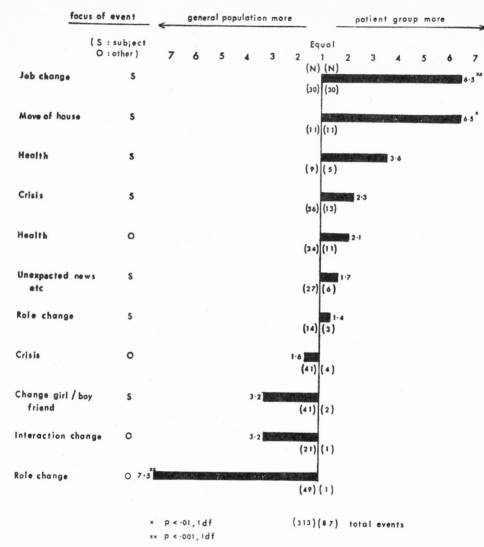

Figure X-1. Schizophrenic and general population ratios of rates of different types of events in a three-month period by whether subject-focused or not.

If the patient and comparison sample are assumed to be comparable in composition, the rate of events in the patient group should not fall *below* that of the general population. A *greater* frequency of a particular type of event among patients can be explained by the events bringing about the disorder and therefore having greater chance of inclusion in the study because patients are selected because of a recent onset. There is no comparable argument to explain lower rates unless we accept the unlikely assumption that certain types of event are negatively related to those producing onset.

Three classes of event were in fact *less* common in the patient groups: "change in opposite-sex friends," "interaction change" due to the movement of others and "role change of others" (Fig. X-1). The latter difference was particularly great.* Patients were expected to have many fewer changes in opposite-sex friends in view of the well-recognized lower marriage rate, especially of men, both before and after the onset of schizophrenic symptoms.[4] The two other differences may well be due to a number of artifacts and be of no particular significance. For example, the lesser frequency of "role changes in others" in the schizophrenic group is at least partly due to the following factors: (1) the patients had somewhat fewer close relatives to whom such incidents could occur; (2) a third fewer close relatives were seen by patients in the previous year; for example, they saw 70 percent of their living children and siblings compared with 88 percent for the general population group, and (3) finally, there was some bias due to the method of selecting women in the general population sample; almost half were interviewed during September and October and this meant that many more children of these women started or left school than would have been the case if the interviews had been spread over the whole year.

A very wide variety of life events therefore appear capable of provoking an acute schizophrenic attack, although events tend to involve directly the patient as the focus of the event. Events also cover a wide spectrum of severity, ranging from death of a close relative to a voluntary change of residence. Recently we have gone over our material and rated each event on the long-term threatening implications scale developed for the depressive study. While many more of the patients than expected from the general population survey had a "markedly" or "moderately" threatening event in the three weeks

---

*"Role change of others" for the general population group consists of: engagement/marriage plans/marriage of siblings (N = 10) and children (N = 11); pregnancy of daughter (N = 4); birth of first child of generation to sibling or child (N = 4); employment change of father/husband in household (N = 8); child starting/leaving school (N = 9), and miscellaneous changes (N = 3).

before onset (28% and 5%, respectively), a large number had events of "some" or "little or no" threatening implications only (32% and 15%, respectively). At least when judged in terms of common sense notions of what is distressing, schizophrenic patients react to a wide range of life events. Of course, the patients may have experienced the events differently, but the results are unlikely to be due to shortcomings in the scale itself. As will be seen, this same scale is extremely successful as an analytical tool in the case of depressive patients. Finally, onset appears to be rarely, if ever, influenced by events occurring outside the three weeks immediately before onset.

DEPRESSIVE RESULTS

The overall results for the depressed patients were similar to those from the schizophrenic study. On average a nine-month period was covered before onset. In the three weeks immediately before onset 51 percent of patients compared with 17 percent of the community had at least one event (p < .001).* Outside the three weeks the rate was very much the same in the two groups and over this period as a whole (i.e. 35 weeks) the difference was not statistically significant.

However, a quite different picture emerges when severity of threatening implications is taken into account. Markedly threatening events are much more common in the *whole period* for the patients than in the community sample. Forty-two percent of the patients had at least one markedly severe event in the period before onset (i.e. 38 weeks). The proportion having such an event in the community in a comparable period was 13 percent (p < .001).† Although there is a greater rate of these events in the three weeks before onset, there is a difference throughout the rest of the period suggesting that the effect of many of the events was not felt for some time.

*The following points should be noted: (a) the 16 percent of the community sample suffering from a clear psychiatric disorder have been *excluded* from all comparisons in this section; (b) results do not change at all when cases with some uncertainty in the dating of onset and events are excluded, and (c) the factors shown to correlate with rate of events among the 325 persons from the community in the schizophrenic study were size of living group and age;[5] as the distribution of these factors was almost the same for depressed patients and the comparison series, we have not applied controls; (d) the period before onset covered for patients ranged between 13 and 52 weeks with an average of 38 weeks.

†Thirty-five male patients were also seen and 54 percent of them had at least one markedly threatening event in the same period before onset.

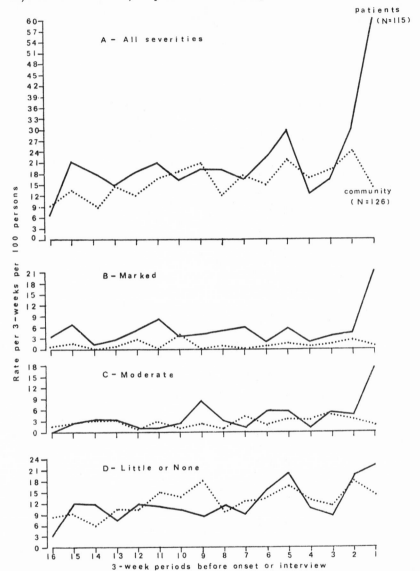

Figure X-2. Rate of events in the 16 three-week periods before onset (patients) or interview (community) by severity of threat.

Since there is little sign of falloff over the whole of the period studied, markedly threatening events could well play a part in the development of the disorder when occurring more than nine months before onset.

TABLE X-II. RATE OF EVENTS FOR A THIRTY-EIGHT WEEK PERIOD FOR DEPRESSED PATIENTS (N = 114) AND A COMPARISON GROUP (N = 185) BY SEVERITY OF THREATENING COMPLICATIONS AND WHETHER EVENT SUBJECT-FOCUSED

	Marked		Moderate		Minor		None	
	Patients	*Comparison*	*Patients*	*Comparison*	*Patients*	*Comparison*	*Patients*	*Comparison*
Subject-focused	.38	.07*	.38	.14*	.41	.38	.60	.60
Nonsubject-focused	.33	.10*	.18	.17	.17	.23	.37	.39
Overall	.71	.17*	.56	.31*	.58	.61	.97	.99

*Difference significant, p < .001

The results for moderately threatening events show a small difference which is restricted to the three weeks before onset. Fifteen percent of the patients compared with 2 percent of the comparison group had such an event in the three weeks (p < .01). Outside the three weeks before onset, however, the rates for the two groups are the same.

There is no difference even in the three weeks before onset between patient and comparison group for events of some or little or no threatening implications and there is, therefore, unlike the schizophrenic study, no suggestion that these more minor events that form three quarters of all events occurring in the general population play any causal role at all.

Some of the other descriptive ratings made for each event can be expected to add to this picture. For instance, a clear-cut result is obtained if in addition to the threatening implications scale we consider whether the event is subject-focused or not (Table X-II). Markedly threatening events are important regardless of the focus of the event. For moderately threatening events 71 percent are subject-focused for the patient and 46 percent for the community sample (p < .01). Subject-focused moderate events are clearly important, whereas there is no evidence that nonsubject-focused moderate events play any role in onset (Table X-II). Nor does this analysis by focus of event alter our earlier conclusion that events of a lesser degree of severity play no role in onset of depression.

The distribution over the period before onset of moderately threatening subject-focused events is similar to the patterning of events found for markedly threatening events. Although these moderate events are much more common in the three weeks immediately prior to onset they also occur more frequently in the remaining nine months before onset.

To summarize these results: 61 percent of patients have at least one markedly threatening or moderately threatening subject-focused event in an average period of thirty-eight weeks before onset, compared with 21 percent in the comparison group. To simplify discussion I will refer to these events as *severe*.

The pattern of results is therefore quite different from that which emerged from the schizophrenic study. Only events with severely threatening implications are causally implicated in the onset of depression. Moreover, although the three-week period immediately before onset contains a particularly large proportion of such events, the rate of these events is also higher for at least the nine months before onset. This is particularly clear for markedly threatening events and the influence of such marked events may indeed last even longer than the period we studied (for example, if we went back eighteen months prior to onset, there still might be a higher rate of marked events).

So far only a part of the material describing each event has been systematically analyzed, but it is already clear that events involved in provoking onset of depression are frequently concerned with some form of "loss." We use this term in a broad sense to include: (1) separation or threat of it, such as death of a parent, or a husband saying he is going to leave home; (2) an unpleasant revelation about someone close forcing a major reassessment of the person and relationship, such as finding out about a husband's unfaithfulness; (3) a life-threatening illness to someone close; (4) a major material loss or disappointment or threat of this, such as a couple living in poor housing learning that their chances of being rehoused were minimal; (5) an enforced change of residence or the threat of it, and, finally, (6) a miscellaneous group of crises involving some element of loss, such as being redundant in a job held for some time or obtaining a legal separation.

Table X-III gives a detailed description of such losses or threats of loss for severe events. Seventy-seven percent of patients with a severely threatening event had at least one of these forms of loss; and loss is therefore much the most important component of long-term threat.

Results for schizophrenic patients as one might expect are different. Of patients who have an event in the three weeks before onset, no more than 30 percent (9/30) have a "loss" event as broadly defined in this study. Three were deaths (father, brother and pet dog); three were enforced changes of residence; two were life-threatening illnesses to someone close, and one was a disappointment over a claim for legal damages because of a minor accident at work.

SOME PRACTICAL IMPLICATIONS

These results from the two studies have important practical implications, and I want to mention these briefly before discussing their theoretical significance. When no distinction is made in terms of

TABLE X-III. PERCENT OF EVENTS AMONG DEPRESSED PATIENTS AND COMPARISON GROUP BY DESCRIPTIVE TYPES AND SEVERITY OF THREATENING IMPLICATIONS

	Markedly Threatening		Moderately Threatening & Subject-Focused		Total	
	Patient	Comparison	Patient	Comparison	Patient	Comparison
Number of events	82	61	44	49	126	110
Type of Event						
1. Separation or major negative revelation about someone close	46[a]	31	23	20	37	26
2. Life-threatening illness to subject	7	10	0	0	5	5
3. Other health crisis to subject	0	0	18	16	6	7
4. Life-threatening illness to someone close	18	25	0	0	11	14
5. Material loss or disappointment or threat of these	7[b]	10	9	4	8	7
6. Crisis in a long-term difficulty	15[c]	11	16	12	15	12
7. Major role change or decision	1	0	25[d]	22	10	10
8. Enforced change of residence or threat of this	0	3	7	12	2	7
9. Miscellaneous crisis	5[e]	10	2	12	4	11
Total	100	100	100	100	100	100
"Loss" events, i.e. 1, 4, 5 and 8	71	69	39	36	58	54

Examples of ratings: [a]Learning that husband having an affair; that child is educationally subnormal.
[b]Learning arrangements for moving from poor housing have failed.
[c]Birth of a child while living in grossly overcrowded conditions.
[d]Leaving home to go to London to join Salvation Army.
[e]Induced abortion in unmarried girl.

severity of the event, then in both schizophrenic and depressive studies a difference between patient and comparison groups would not have been found without careful attention to the dating of events and onset, and subsequent detailed specification of the length of the time period to be studied before onset. Ideally, events and onset should be dated to within one week of their occurrence. When all events are considered, large differences emerged in both studies in the rate of events in the three-week period immediately before onset; this difference, however, largely disappears when longer periods are taken. For example, in the schizophrenic study the difference is greatly reduced if a thirteen-week period before onset is taken (the rate per 100 people was 174 and 96 in patient and comparison groups), and it can be calculated that the difference would largely disappear if twelve months were taken (estimate of 462 and 384 per 100, respectively). When events are characterized in terms of severity of long-term threat, the same argument applies to events of moderate severity in both studies and to events of little or no severity in the schizophrenic study.

This is not so for marked (or moderate subject-focused) events as is most clearly seen in the depressive study. Such a reduction does not occur if the event is rare in the community sample; indeed, so long as there is a raised rate in the patient group for the whole of the period taken, lengthening the period will increase the size of the difference. Further, the exact dating of events in the period is not critical; in the depressive study it would have been enough to establish whether or not the patient had a severely threatening event in the nine months before onset.

Thus, an investigator can reduce his chance of obtaining a positive result in two ways: if he does not pay close attention to the dating of events relative to onset he is unlikely to establish the kind of result found in the schizophrenic study, and if he does not differentiate events by some measure of severity he cannot establish the kind of result found with severely threatening events in the depressive study. For example, a recent study has emphasized the significance of its failure to find clear-cut relations between life events and the onset of various psychiatric conditions.[12] However, the study neither closely dated onset and events nor rated events by some measure of severity. This, plus the use of a physically ill comparison group, may well account for its largely negative results.[9]

THE NATURE OF THE CAUSAL LINK BETWEEN
LIFE EVENTS AND ONSET OF PSYCHIATRIC CONDITIONS

We believe that results from the two London studies and the work of others on the role of life changes and crises in the onset of psychiatric disorders indicate that a serious case can now be made for the importance of such events in several pathological conditions.[10,14-16,18,21] This is so in spite of difficult methodological problems which, as we have argued elsewhere, can be largely overcome.[9] However, just what kind of causal role these life events have and whether this role differs for schizophrenic and depressive patients still remains for discussion.

In evaluating individual patients most psychiatrists will agree that life events often seem of importance, but many will then go on to say that they merely aggravate a pre-existing condition or assert that constitutional or other bodily influences must be the major etiological factors because so many people experience such events without breaking down.[19] On the whole the matter is not dealt with much better in the scientific literature; it is almost always allowed to rest once a case has been made for some kind of causal effect. The concept of predisposition is clearly central, which traditionally involves genetic and constitutional differences, early childhood experiences and personality traits; it is also feasible when dealing with the role of life events to take account of ongoing social difficulties and amount of current social support as part of the predispositional nexus. Although there seems at present little hope of dealing all at once with such a host of possible influences in a satisfactory manner, it is possible to come to some conclusions about the nature of the causal link involved. My colleagues and I have discussed the matter in detail elsewhere and I will summarize our main argument only.[7]

The significance of an event might range from simply triggering a disorder, which was about to occur in any case, to a situation where it is of *formative* importance. The first view emphasizes the importance of predispositional factors and plays down the influence of life events. Events are seen as triggering an illness that would probably have occurred before long for other reasons and at most may bring onset forward by a short period of time. The opposing view is that events play an important role, and onset is either substantially advanced in time by the event or brought about by it altogether. Consideration of the schizophrenic and depressive results from a theoretical perspective, we believe, can throw light on this fundamental issue and allow us to make a choice between the two positions for a particular set of results.

For the purposes of this paper I shall refer to any onset not brought about by an observed event as "spontaneous" even though the onset might be due to an unobserved event or social factors such as long-term difficulties, loneliness and the like. The model we have developed views each person as having an overall onset rate for a particular psychiatric condition. Onset rate refers to the probability of onset of occurrence in a short period of time and has two components, one stemming from the influence of particular life events and one from a spontaneous process. In our depressive study the latter includes any influence not arising from life events occurring in the twelve-month period prior to onset.

Thus, a person might have a chance of developing a disorder starting in adolescence which increases slightly as he grows older but which is much increased after his mother's death when he is thirty. We assume that after such an event there is a definite probability that it will cause an onset, although the onset itself may not follow for months or even years. However, for any one person we cannot establish whether an onset was "provoked" or "spontaneous" since we have no idea of the spontaneous rate for any one individual; but it is relatively simple to calculate for a group of patients the proportion of onsets that were provoked by events in a defined period before onset.

I shall refer to the proportion of provoked onsets as x—it is simply the proportion of patients having at least one event in a fixed period before onset minus the proportion of onsets where one would expect onset and event to be juxtaposed by chance. This is easily done and the reduction in the original proportion will usually be small.

We believe that it follows (if the view I have outlined is accepted) that in the study of life events we must estimate both (1) the proportion of onsets that have been brought about by events (x), and (2) the average time after such a provoked onset when a spontaneous onset would otherwise have occurred. This second estimate, the time from provoked to spontaneous onset, is the critical measure for our present purpose and we call it the *brought forward time*.

The brought forward time is a minimal estimate of the average length of time between onset provoked by an event and spontaneous onset had no event occurred. We base our calculations of this time on a number of assumptions which we show lead to a conservative estimate. We call it the brought forward time because we believe that it gives an estimate of the average time events have brought forward onset. Its length is greater the rarer the event is in the general population and the greater the proportion of patients with an event. The estimate of the brought forward time, we believe, is so conservative that we do not interpret the estimate itself literally, but its length does allow us to choose between the two rival causal hypotheses, and it was for this that it was designed. If it is long, say one year, we believe that a triggering effect is untenable. It is incompatible with our definition of such an effect as bringing about an illness that probably would have occurred before long anyway. Therefore, if the time given is implausibly long, a formative effect is indicated.

Since we have described elsewhere in detail our method of calculating the brought forward time, I will here only give an outline. Two empirical measures are needed. For the first, the proportion of patients with an event leading to onset, I have already mentioned that it is necessary to make a correction to the proportion with one or more events within some fixed period before onset to take account of the possible juxtaposition by chance of onset and event. This corrected proportion I have referred to as x. The reduction will usually be relatively small. Second, it is necessary to know the usual rate of life events for persons such as patients outside the period involved in the illness. The rate in the patient group itself cannot be taken because, as patients have been specially selected for study because of a recent onset, they will be bound to have a high rate of events if there is any causal link between the two. This can be illustrated by considering two ways of calculating the frequency (or rate) of heavy drinking among drivers of cars. One way would be to find out how long before a car accident a driver had taken a large quantity of alcohol. Another would be to select the same people at some random point in their lives and find out when they last drank heavily. It is clear that two quite different rates would be obtained. Since it is known that drinking is related to car accidents, selecting individuals because of a car accident would mean that the time between heavy drinking and the point of interview would be much less than in the random time sampling. This distinction is so important for our argument that we label the two rates differently: (1) the measure obtained by random sampling which, we believe, accurately reflects the rate of heavy drinking among drivers of cars and which we call *the true rate*, and (2) that obtained by measuring backwards in time from a car accident which we call the *conditional rate*. If there is a causal link, this conditional rate cannot, under any circumstances, be used to reflect the true rate; this is the situation with severely threatening events and the onset of depression. The true rate of such events can be based on the rate well before onset, on the rate obtained in a follow-up study some time after onset, or on the rate in a matched group of randomly selected individuals in the community from which the patients were drawn. We use the latter estimate based on the *total* community sample irrespective of whether sample members were psychiatrically disturbed (i.e. for this estimate we now include the 16 percent of women who were rated as showing definite psychiatric disturbance in the community sample of the depressive study). I will call this estimate of the true rate the *patient life event rate*.

Next we need to estimate, on the basis of our theoretical assumptions, the average time from an onset produced by an event to the time when a spontaneous onset would have occurred had no events intervened (which we call the brought forward time).

I will take a simplified example to illustrate the kind of argument we employ. To obtain an estimate of the brought forward time we must obtain some estimate of the spontaneous onset rate near the time of observed onset. Let us suppose that we have calculated the proportion of onsets provoked by a life event and found it is one-third. The proportion of onsets that occurred spontaneously is thus two-thirds, so the ratio of provoked to spontaneous is 1 to 2. We can take this to equal the ratio of provoked onset *rate* to spontaneous onset *rate*. Therefore to obtain the spontaneous onset rate we only need to find the one unknown in the equation, the provoked onset rate.* This cannot be directly measured, but an estimate can

*Ie. $\dfrac{\text{proportion with a provoked onset}}{\text{proportion with a spontaneous onset}} = \dfrac{\text{provoked onset rate}}{\text{spontaneous onset rate}}$

be made indirectly, using the conservative assumption that all events of the type under consideration lead to onset. Under this assumption the provoked onset rate is the same as the patient life event rate, as each life event is assumed to be accompanied by an onset. Since, in our example, the ratio of provoked onset rate to spontaneous onset rate is 1 to 2, the frequency of spontaneous onsets is double the patient life event rate. On average, therefore, each patient's expected time to next spontaneous onset from any point in time will be half his expected time to next life event. The latter can be obtained from the total community sample. Since we are measuring from the point of onset, this expected time to next spontaneous onset for a patient whose onset was provoked is the time by which provoking events "brought forward" his onset. This is precisely the brought forward time which we seek, i.e. the average distance from a provoked onset to when a spontaneous onset would otherwise have occurred. It may be that there is a substantial delay between a life event and the onset which it causes; we refer to this as a long-term influence.[1] However, whatever the length of time between event and onset, the brought forward time is still measured from the time of provoked onset, not event, and the result is unaffected.

Let me mention some results. Those for the schizophrenic study support a triggered effect: the brought forward time is on average ten weeks. The depressive result for markedly threatening events equally unequivocably support a formative effect: the brought forward time is on average two years. The brought forward time for moderately threatening subject-focused events in the depressive study is just over one year, again suggesting that formative effect is operative. Thirty-five percent of the patients had such an event in the thirty-eight weeks before onset and in just over half of these (19%) it was not associated with a markedly threatening event. Thus, allowing for the correction I have already mentioned that takes account of the chance juxtaposition of event and onset, about half the depressive patients had an event causally linked with onset which in most cases seems likely to have been of formative importance.

FINAL COMMENTS

A final conclusion about the proportion of depressed patients involved in some kind of environmental effect cannot be established until we have fully analyzed our material concerning other environmental factors such as long-term difficulties and amount of social support. Such factors may well interact in some way with life events or act independently to produce the disorder. In the schizophrenic work we have spent a good deal of time investigating such long-term influences. Three separate studies have indicated that the nature of the home environment plays a powerful role in determining whether a discharged schizophrenic patient will relapse in the following year with florid symptoms.[3, 6, 8] The results concerning life events suggest in the light of this work that for schizophrenic patients most life events seem to trigger the onset of florid symptoms in those who are not only predisposed to the condition, but are experiencing tense and difficult situations at home (probably also this would hold for difficult relations at work or in some key relationship outside the home). It is also possible that for some persons events may be sufficiently traumatic to bring about onset without the experience of such ongoing "arousing" situations. Sixteen percent of the schizophrenic patients did have a markedly threatening event in the three months before onset, a proportion much greater than expected, but the results of our brought forward index do not allow us to conclude that a formative effect was involved.

Analysis so far of the depressive material suggests a radically different picture. Since we found 16 percent of the women in the community were suffering from a definite psychiatric disorder, most with a clear depressive element, genetic and other background factors probably play a much smaller role. Moreover, we have shown that life events are largely of formative importance. This as yet is a preliminary analysis. We also have, for example, material on ongoing difficulties that have not been brought about by a life event occurring in the year. They also play some role in onset but it is too early to tell in what way this differs from that of schizophrenic patients. Although preliminary, the results underline the importance of distinguishing broad diagnostic groups in this kind of research; this does not mean that finer distinctions will be found useful, however. An exhaustive analysis of symptomatology in our work on schizophrenic patients showed no evidence that our results concerning life events or the role of interpersonal relations in the home applied to particular subgroups of schizophrenic patients.[2,6] We have yet to analyze such detailed clinical material in the depressive study. However, I think it is reasonable to conclude that a research worker ignores diagnostic factors at his peril in the study of life events and onset of psychiatric disorders.

REFERENCES

1. Antonovsky, A.: Breakdown: A needed fourth step in the conceptual armamentarium of modern medicine. Presented at the First International Conference of Social Science and Medicine, Aberdeen, Scotland, September 4-6, 1968.
2. Birley, J.L.T., and Brown, G.W.: Crises and life changes preceding the onset or relapse of acute schizophrenia: clinical aspects. *Br J Psychiatr, 116*:327-333, 1970.
3. Brown, G.W.: Experiences of discharged chronic schizophrenic patients in various types of living group. *Milbank Memorial Fund Q, 37*:105-131, 1959.
4. ————: The family of the schizophrenic patient. In Coppen, A.J. and Walk, A. (Eds.): *Recent Developments in Schizophrenia: A Symposium.* London, Royal Medico-Psychological Association, 1967.
5. ————, and Birley, J.L.T.: Crises and life changes and the onset of schizophrenia. *J Health Soc Behav, 9*:302-314, 1968.
6. ————, Birley, J.L.T., and Wing, J.K.: The influence of family life on the course of schizophrenic illness: A replication. *Br J Psychiatr, 121*:241-258, 1972.
7. ————, Harris, T.O., and Peto, J.: Life events and psychiatric disorders: 2. Nature of causal link. *Psychol Med,* In press.
8. ————, Monck, E., Carstairs, G.M., and Wing, J.K.: The influence of family life on the course of schizophrenic illness. *Br J Prev Soc Med, 16*:55-68, 1962.
9. ————, Sklair, F., Harris, T.O., and Birley, J.L.T.: Life events and psychiatric disorders: 1. Some methodological issues. *Psychol Med, 3*:74-87, 1973.
10. Cooper, B., and Shepherd, M.: Life change, stress and mental disorder: The ecological approach. In Harding, John (Ed.): *Recent Advances in Psychological Medicine.* London, Butterworth, 1970.
11. Faris, R.E., and Dunham, H.W.: *Mental Disorders in Urban Areas.* Chicago, University of Chicago Press, 1939.
12. Hudgens, R.W., Robins, E., and Deland, W.B.: The reporting of recent stress in the lives of psychiatric patients. *Br J Psychiatr, 117*:635-643, 1970.
13. Gove, W.G.: Societal reaction as an explanation of mental illness: An evaluation. *Am Soc Rev, 35*:873-883, 1970.
14. Parkes, C.M.: Recent bereavement as a cause of mental illness. *Br J Psychiatr, 110*:198-204, 1964.

15. Paykel, E.S.: Life events and depression. Presented at the annual meeting of the American Association for the Advancement of Science, Chicago, Illinois, December 26-30, 1970.
16. ————, Myers, J.K., Dienelt, M.N., Klerman, G.L., Lindenthal, J.J., and Pepper, M.P.: Life events and depression: A controlled study. *Arch Gen Psychiatr, 21*:753-760, 1969.
17. Rahe, R.H.: Life crisis and health change. In May, P.R.A., and Wittenborn, J.R. (Eds.): *Psychotropic Drug Response: Advances in Prediction.* Springfield, Ill., Thomas, 1969.
18. Reid, D.D.: Precipitating proximal factors in the occurrence of mental disorders: Epidemiological evidence. *Milbank Memorial Fund Q, 39*: 227-248, 1961.
19. Russell-Davis, D.: Depression as adaptation to crises. *Br J Med Psychol, 43*:109-116, 1970.
20. Scheff, T.: *Being Mentally Ill.* Chicago, Aldine Press, 1966.
21. Steinberg, H.R., and Durell, J.: A stressful situation as a precipitant of schizophrenic symptoms. *Br J Psychiatr, 114*:1097-1105, 1968.
22. Syme, S.L.: Implications and future prospects. In Syme, S.L., and Reeder, L.G. (Eds.): Social stress and cardiovascular disease. *Milbank Memorial Fund Q, 45*:175-180, Part 2, 1967.
23. Szasz, T.S.: *The Myth of Mental Illness.* London, Secker and Worburg, 1961.
24. Wing, J.K., Birley, J.L.T., Cooper, J.E., Graham, P., and Isaacs, A.D.: Reliability of procedure for measuring and classifying "present psychiatric state." *Br J Psychiatr, 113*:499-515, 1967.
25. Ziegler, E., and Phillips, L.: Psychiatric diagnosis: A critique. *J Abnorm Soc Psychol, 63*:607-618, 1961.

Chapter XI

STRESSFUL FACTORS IN GREEK LIFE LEADING TO ILLNESS

C. S. Ierodiakonou, N. Kokantzis and L. Fekas

G REEK SOCIETY may be considered as basically a Western society, though due to the geographical position of Greece in the southeast of Europe and its prolonged occupation by the Ottoman Empire, it still retains certain oriental cultural aspects in its structure. These render a rather unique character to the Greek way of life, still evident mainly in the small towns and villages. The postwar period, with the influx of tourists, the spread of mass communication media, the increased contact with Western ideas and their influence, has started a rapidly accelerating change, which has, naturally, manifested itself first and foremost in the capital and big towns but much less so, as yet, in the rural areas. However, the family remains the most important social unit; it is closely knit and has an extended character which contains often up to three generations.

We here propose to examine some of the social factors which have an effect on the psychological development of the individual in Greece and some of which have been found to lead to stress and illness. It would probably offer a clearer picture if we started by studying the various periods of life in their chronological sequence, that is, from childhood onwards through adolescence and maturity to old age.

In regard to child rearing and, in particular, breast feeding, a study by Vassiliou and Vassiliou[10] has revealed that the great majority of Greek mothers continue to breast feed their children

(90% compared with 39% of American mothers) but tend to show a differential treatment in favor of boys. This reflects the still prevailing attitude in Greek families to place sons on a more privileged footing than girls, which could be explained by the fact that the son used to be, and to some extent still is, the future leader and supporter of the family, the "fighter," the carrier of the family name, whereas the girl is a much more dependent member of the family until the time of her marriage. Even then, in fact, it is still customary for her family to provide her with a dowry.

Concerning toilet training, it appears that it tends to last a little longer in Greece than in the U.S.A., and again boys seem to receive preferential treatment in that their training starts and ends earlier than that of the girls. Thus, the average age of starting is nine months for the boys and twelve months for the girls. Regarding the parental attitude on discipline in general, it appears that this may be quite demanding but also rather inconsistent, alternating between pampering and punishment, according to the parental mood of the moment. It should be pointed out here that children in Greece play an important role in the family prestige. Parents expect them to be exemplary in their behavior and achievement and thus bring honor to the family. As we shall see later, this attitude persists during adolescence and even adulthood and often proves a very stressful psychological factor.

Sexual education of children is considered a delicate matter on which Greek parents, in the majority, are still rather reluctant to dwell. As Kokantzis and Ierodiakonou found in a study of anxiety patients,[6] a great majority of them did not have an enlightened attitude towards sexual life, due to the inhibiting influence of their training and the strict moral, religious and social conventions which still largely prevail in Greek society. These patients, therefore, had to suppress their sexual drives to the point of denying the existence of the problem and appearing superficially indifferent or asexual. In the writers' experience, in spite of the fact that coitus interruptus is widely practiced in the rural areas of Greece as a measure of birth control, the problem is not, as Freud considered, one of physical satisfaction and physiological discharge, but is due to the inability of these patients to feel free to have sexual intercourse.

According to other studies[8] the parent-child roles in Greece involve greater affection and less rejection than in America. The highest respect is found in the mother-son relationship. In the father-son relationship, the father is the one to punish insubordination yet he is perceived only in a controlling and not in a commanding position. The son asks for help but also usually fears the father. There is no role demand for the son to express affection towards the father. To quote, "The mother is perceived as giving positive affection to the son, admiration and assistance, and the son responds equally with positive affection and subordination, expressing gratitude and admiration."[8]

Overprotection has often been found to go together with constant inhibiting criticism of behavior. The parents often expect too much of their children, thus pushing them beyond their abilities and their own inclinations. Under such conditions a child will probably reach adolescence with a number of defects, such as early fixations, incomplete synthesizing functions, poorly integrated and internalized value system, and disturbed self-identity, as is confirmed by clinical examination according to Vassiliou.[9]

Similar stressful factors were found in a study by Ierodiakonou on the psychological problems of Greek University students.[1] It is noteworthy that most of the subjects of this study developed their neurotic or psychosomatic symptoms in the period just before and during their first year in the University. These were usually young people who were greatly dependent on their families and had difficulty in leaving home and being on their own, especially when this meant moving from a small village into a big town "among unknown people." This is typical of the close intrafamilial relations in Greece. In fact, there were many cases where the dependency on their mother was so marked that the symptoms subsided whenever these students had an opportunity of revisiting their homes. In this connection, it must be pointed out that the quite sharp differences in principles and attitudes between the strict mentality of village life and the much more liberal one of the big town, which still characterize Greek society, often prove a very stressful factor for the young student who is faced with the dilemma of moral choice. This was supported by the fact that the greater number of students with neurotic symptoms came from the School of Theology and Philosophy.

Another stage during which a high frequency of symptoms was observed was towards the end of their university studies and the obtaining of their degrees. This meant for them that they now had to face life on their own, to take on new responsibilities, and, far from being supported economically by their families, to become now themselves the providers.

Another problem which the young adult has now to face is often the arrangement and solution of his sexual and love affairs. Marriage is still considered in Greece as the only acceptable and honorable form of relation between a man and a woman and to which a love affair should ultimately lead. On the other hand, the achievement of professional and financial security are not easily available to the average Greek who has a hard struggle ahead of him before he can feel ready to start his own family. He has to support his old parents and often to provide for the dowry of his unmarried sisters, if any, as is still the cultural custom in Greece. All these reasons explain why men in Greece often marry much later than in more developed Western countries—though this situation is now steadily improving with the rising of living standards.

This brings us to the problems of people who become parents at an advanced age.[2] The psychological needs to have children, which in fact express the wish for continuation of one's self and, especially in Greece, of one's family name, as well as for security and support in old age, are felt much more keenly by people who are already in an advanced age and who, therefore, await with increasing anxiety the arrival of the first child. The age at which they become parents will influence their attitudes toward their children. It is possible that it will mean a greater consistency of behavior and care, but it may also result in a rigidity of views and attitudes on the part of the parents who find it difficult to see eye to eye with their children. When the children eventually grow up, these differences often result in a clash between them. By the time the child has become an adolescent, the parent, and especially the father (husbands tend very often to be much older than their wives in Greece), is an old man. The differences become more acute, the child regards the parent as an "anachronism," and discipline and respect are greatly diminished. As Ierodiakonou found in his study,[2] many of these children become delinquents.

The mental problems, and especially anxiety and neurotic traits, of old age have been examined in two studies by Ierodiakonou, Kokantzis and Routsoni.[5,7] The following findings were observed: no essential difference was found in the level of manifest anxiety between old age and younger groups, though it should be mentioned here that, on the whole, the level of anxiety of the Greek population sample is considerably higher than that of corresponding American and British norms. Women were constantly proved to be more anxiety-prone than men, even more so than in other countries, probably due to the specific Greek cultural factors. Neurotic traits were found much more frequently in the older age groups than in the younger ones, characterized especially by depressive and submissive tendencies. Nevertheless, suicidal attempts among the aged were observed much less frequently (15% of the total attempts) compared with the statistics of other Western countries.[3] This should be attributed to the supportive role of the family within which old people in Greece are expected to spend the remainder of their lives.

Apart from the aforementioned stressful factors leading to illness, the Greek patient has to face the prejudices and misconceptions which characterize the attitude of the general public towards mental illness.[4]

REFERENCES

1. Ierodiakonou, C.S.: Some psychopathological mechanisms of Greek university students seen in an outpatient service. Presented at the 15th Meeting of the European League for Mental Hygiene, in Athens, Greece, 1965.

2. ————: Psychological reactions of people who have become parents at an advanced age. (Greek text.) *Galenus, 10*:577-585, 1968.

3. ————, Dimitriou, E., and Partsaphyllides, T.: Suicide attempts in Thessaloniki area: Clinical and psychopathological findings of the first year of research. Presented at the IV International Congress of Social Psychiatry, in Jerusalem, May 1972.

4. ————, and Routsoni, A.: An investigation of the attitudes toward the mentally handicapped in a section of the Greek public. Proc frm Annual Meeting of the European League of Ment Hlth, held in Istanbul, 1969, pp. 108-116.

5. ————, Routsoni, A., and Kokantzis, N.: Neurotic trends in certain groups of pre-senile and senile subjects, investigated through the I.P.A.T. *Acta Neurol Psychiatr Hell, 8*:25-33, 1969. (Greek text.)

6. Kokantzis, N., and Ierodiakonou, C.S.: Characteristics of anxiety states in Greek patients. Proc frm IV World Congress of Psychiatry, held

in Madrid, 1966, pp. 1470-1472.

7. Routsoni, A., Ierodiakonou, C.S., and Kokantzis, N.: Manifest anxiety level in certain groups of pre-senile and senile subjects through the I.P.A.T. anxiety scale. *Acta Neurol Psychiatr Hell,* 7:253-263, 1968. (Greek text.)

8. Triandis, H., Vassiliou, V., and Nassiakou, M.: Some cross-cultural studies of subjective culture. Technical Report No. 45, Urbana, Ill. Group Effectiveness Laboratory, 1967.

9. Vassiliou, G.: Aspects of parent-adolescent transaction in the Greek family. In Caplan, G., and Lebovici, S. (Eds.): *The Adolescent: Psychosocial Perspectives.* New York, Basic Books, 1969.

10. ————, and Vassiliou, V.: On aspects of child-rearing in Greece. In Anthony, E. James (Ed.): *The Child in His Family.* New York, Wiley & Sons, 1970.

Chapter XII

EXTREME STRESS IN ADULT LIFE AND ITS PSYCHIC AND PSYCHOPHYSIOLOGICAL CONSEQUENCES

Ransom J. Arthur

Between 1815 and 1914, although there were localized conflicts in the Crimea in 1854, and three Prussian wars with Denmark, Austria and France in 1864, 1866 and 1870, respectively, there was no general and protracted war in Europe. It was in this relatively pacific climate that Professor Freud was born in 1856.[21-23] Although his childhood was marked by the Austro-Prussian War, in fact, that war was of very brief duration. It is quite understandable in view of the era in which he grew up that in the evolution of his professional thought, he initially gave little weight to factors involving aggression, hatred, cruelty and destructiveness. In fact, among many other reasons, the actual theoretical quarrel between Professor Freud and Alfred Adler, so well documented in the Minutes of the Vienna Psycho-Analytic Society in the years 1907 and 1908, which eventually led to Adler's leaving the Psycho-Analytic movement, dealt with the emphasis that Alfred Adler placed upon the role of aggression in human life.[29,30]

At that period Freud felt, first, that all adult neuroses had as their precursors childhood neuroses, and that the basis of all neuroses was sexual vicissitudes rather than aggressive or destructive conflicts. However, in August 1914, Europe began a cataclysmic general war.

At the time the war began, Freud's reactions were those of other patriotic Austrians of his class. In fact, his sons served in the Austro-Hungarian forces. But, as the years rolled on to 1918, the full horror of this conflict gradually revealed itself. The enormous destructiveness could not help but impinge upon his professional thinking. He then recognized the existence of the traumatic neuroses of war in which childhood precursors of illness were difficult to discern.

The celebrated cases which appear in Freud's earlier writings, those of Little Hans, Wolfman, Ratman, Dora, Elizabeth von R., etc., were all of young people. In all those individuals the primary influence of childhood problems upon the development of their neuroses was apparent. But now, during the course of the First World War, Freud corresponded with, amongst others, Karl Abraham, his distinguished colleague who, with Freud, developed the classical psychoanalytic theory of the etiology of depression.

Karl Abraham was a medical officer with the German Army and had frequent professional contact with cases of war neuroses. These cases of traumatic neuroses which appeared *de novo* in adult life were obviously connected with horrifying experiences which the patients had undergone during the conflict. Evaluation of his wartime experiences led to a revision of Freud's thinking. In 1919, Freud wrote *Beyond the Pleasure Principle* in which, for the first time, he came to grips with a dark side of human nature, nonerotic, vile in some of its manifestations, but clearly to be recognized if one wished to speak about human behavior and the etiology of the neuroses.[16]

The years following 1919, of course, saw the rise of certain movements of a totalitarian character which eventuated in systematic cruelty of an unprecedented kind. The comprehensiveness and vastness of twentieth century cruelty was truly without precise parallel. Of course, one cannot overlook, in speaking of cruelty, for example, the ancient Romans. Caesar's *Commentaries* contain accounts of virtual genocide of Gallic tribes which opposed him. Similarly, the gladiatorial combat seen at the Colosseum had a kind of naked barbarity that we would find difficult to accept. However, the Romans lacked the scientific and administrative machinery to carry out the crimes of the twentieth century's concentration camps.

But after the First World War, Freud and, indeed during the Second World War as well, after Freud's death, Freudian psychiatrists felt it necessary to postulate a predisposition to traumatic neuroses. They maintained that there were, even among those who broke down in combat or in other circumstances of a similar character, weaknesses of a neurotic type springing from deleterious childhood experiences.[18] It would appear at present that it is unnecessary to put forward predisposition as a *sine qua non* of adult traumatic neuroses. Stereotypic syndromes have appeared in millions of humans subjected to extreme stress, the majority of whom had functioned well prior to the traumatic experiences. The victims of the German concentration camps are a classical case in point.[1, 4, 9]

Following the accession of Hitler to power, he ordered the Reichsfuhrer S. S. Heinrich Himmler to establish concentration camps, that is prisons in which all kinds of prisoners could be placed, particularly those of a political character, a vast array of individuals whom someone suspected of being antipathetic to the regime. Already in the 1930's an enormous number of people were seized at odd hours of the night and carried off to these camps. In 1941, a deliberate governmental policy was established to exterminate all considered to be enemies of the state. This mass slaughter was carried out in a systematic manner and in the case of the Jews, was called "the final solution." A number of fearsome stresses existed in these camps.

Malnutrition was ubiquitous. The rations were always kept at an extremely low level. Crowding was severe. Eight people might have to share what would amount to some kind of a slab. Sleep deprivation was the norm. Exposure to the elements while working was common and the garments provided were always insufficient. Labor was forced. There were beatings and all kinds of other tortures. The prisoners were kept exhausted. Some were experimented upon for what was euphemistically called medical purposes. Various infectious diseases were endemic. There was forced transport or forced marches which added to the overall stress.

In addition to these physical stressors, there was seen nonphysical stress of the most sinister type. There was the real and continuous threat of death. Prisoners seemed to be chosen for execution in the most capricious way. It often depended upon the whims of the guards as to which victim would be chosen at any given point in time. They would appear to mark prisoners for death in a random way. This uncertainty added to the terror. There was separation of family members and humiliation was a daily occurrence. Frustration of all drives took place. Hunger, thirst, sexual drives, even the need for voiding or defecating were unsatisfied under the circumstances. The prisoners, when they were not being brutalized themselves, had to witness all kinds of cruelty. In every way there was an attempt to destroy any sense of human dignity or human identity. In fact, the entire indoctrination was geared to convince the prisoners that they were indeed inferior objects, in every way nonhuman and deserving of what was happening to them. Millions died but many survived by one miracle or another.

There were recognized subcategories among the prisoners. There was a group called in the concentration camps "musselmen" who lost all interest in living and withdrew all interests in the outside world and who died very quickly without obvious cause. The same phenomenon has been described in prisoners of war. Some American prisoners of the Japanese during the Death March from Bataan in the Philippine Islands in 1942 and some subsequently in Korea also exhibited a giving up syndrome. Yet, in virtually every situation there are those who retain an implacable will to survive.

For all, the initial stage of captivity was one of shock, terror and a sense of unreality. Each person felt that it might be a nightmare from which one would awake safe. It was not a nightmare but reality itself. Following the initial stage of shock, regressive behavior appeared, accompanied by extreme dependence and rescue fantasies. In some cases, there was identification with the aggressor, that is, some of the prisoners emulated the behavior of their captors. Denial, of course, was ubiquitous and a principal mechanism of adaptation. Deadening of the emotional life and a constriction or narrowing of concentration were used in an attempt to minimize the horrifying stimuli that were flooding in continuously. Curiously enough the ordinary psychiatric disorders such as the psychoneuroses and the psychoses appeared to diminish in incidence. To become psychotic was to die, of course, because the implacable captors would waste no time with the insane. For many people who survived, incarceration was prolonged. All the while, they cherished fantasies about what the postwar world would be like. They dreamed of avenging the injustices they had seen and of building a bright new life for themselves.

Then came the time of liberation. And with it, still further stress. Life is often not just or equitable and those who had suffered had more travail ahead. Many former prisoners tried to return or returned briefly to their old homes or tried to check up on the relatives and had their worse fears confirmed. Their families had been destroyed during The Holocaust. Some were put in Displaced Persons Camps for considerable periods of time. This further confinement engendered more anger and resentment. They felt that they were once again being mistreated by uncaring authorities. Some of this bitterness arose from the submerged rage which they had not been able to express towards their previous captors. Immediately after the war, a definite phenomenon was described and given the name KZ syndrome (from the German words for concentration camp, *Konzentrationlager*). This syndrome consisted of obvious defects of memory, defects of concentration, and intellectual defects along with a whole host of symptoms such as anxiety, depression and various psychosomatic manifestations.[8,11,12,19]

Then, there was, of course, a fanning out from the camps of the exprisoners. Many emigrated to Israel, to Canada, to the United States of America, to Australia or other nations. Others returned to their homelands.

Extensive reports from Israel, from Canada and from the United States have shown that former prisoners continued to require medical care at a rate much greater than that of the general population.[10,14,25,31] These patients were described as being seclusive, apathetic, socially isolated, passive and dependent. Still others were also described as being suspicious, hostile, bitter and belligerent. Followup studies have been done over the years, partially because of the question of compensation for the exprisoners by the West German government. Compensation probably played a minor role in symptom maintenance. The patients have continued to exhibit anxiety, irritability, restlessness and apprehensiveness, startle reactions, and nightmares. Even after a quarter century, they also show dysphoria, depression, memory loss and difficulty in concentration.

The psychosomatic manifestations particularly involve the gastrointestinal tract with dyspepsia, vague pains, diarrhea, as well as weakness and fatigue. There is often an obsessive ruminative state with much guilt about supposedly unworthy acts committed in the camps. Thus one now sees a relatively uniform syndrome in adults that apparently has resulted from the stress of unprecedented barbarities.

The Norwegians have also reported on syndromes among those who were prisoners of the Nazis.[13, 15, 38] They felt that a group of 227 former prisoners intensively studied was characterized by definite psychic deviations and that 189, or 83 percent, showed the KZ syndrome. The Norwegian workers felt that they could divide this syndrome into two subtypes with differing etiology. The cerebro-organic included memory loss, confusion, difficulty in concentration and losses of intelligence. These manifestations were considered to be due to the severe malnutrition and the ferocious beatings to the head that had been administered. The manifestations of the other category—anxiety, depression and so forth—were considered to be psychic sequelae of the general brutality of the experience.

A recent report from Canada indicates that psychic problems may not be confined to the first generation.[36] The children of parents or a parent who had been in a concentration camp were brought to child guidance clinics with greater frequency than would be expected from the population at risk. Careful study revealed difficulties with the families in several areas. First, as compared to control or comparison families, the concentration camp victims' families had much more difficulty in controlling or disciplining their children. There was also an overevaluation of the children's abilities. The whole theme of discipline and aggression was a forbidden one between the parent and the children. There appeared to be an excessive amount of fighting between the children in one of these families. Sibling rivalry and battles were fierce because the struggles between the generations were muted. The parents showed an intense preoccupation with past events and in the same sense they were partially absent from the home because of the remembrance of what they had undergone and the losses that they had suffered. They had few resources left for coping with the children. Children, of course, resent parental preoccupation and act out in other ways. The children seemed to be on their way to becoming guilt-ridden, depressed adults with imperfect egos. The children felt guilty about making normal demands upon their parents because the patients were so bound up with their past deprivations.

Prisoners of war in this century have also, in some instances, undergone severe stress in adult life.[2,3,6,26,35,41] For the Americans, captivity in Germany was associated with the relatively low death rate of 4 percent. However, among the American prisoners of the Japanese, the death rate ran about 60 percent. Many, many of the stressors of the concentration camps applied to the prisoners of war of the Japanese. There was grossly insufficient food, crowded living conditions, forced labor, capricious cruelty, beatings, everything except indoctrination. The Japanese apparently did not try to indoctrinate the prisoners with enthusiasm for the Greater East Asia Co-prosperity Sphere or All Asia One Culture. The Japanese prisoners of the Americans, on the other hand, were very well treated.

For the years following release from captivity by the Japanese, the death rate for the former prisoners was several times that of a comparison group of servicemen who had not been prisoners.[27] Some of the excess mortality was due to tuberculosis but a large amount of the increase was accounted for by accidents, suicides and homicide. After a decade had passed the death rate fell to that of the general veteran population. English former prisoners of the Japanese also reported excess postwar difficulties.

The Korean War added the element of Communist political indoctrination to the physical and mental cruelties. During the 1930's in Russia, during the time of great Stalinist purges as depicted by the novel *Darkness at Noon* by Arthur Koestler, there was an attempt to indoctrinate all prisoners by allegedly scientific methods by which the prisoner would be brought to a realization that, due to motives of which he had been previously unaware, he had, in fact, been a reactionary or deviationist right along. He was directed by various means to realize his errors, sign a confession, appear in court, be convicted and then executed without remonstrance. During The Great Purge a fantastic percentage of the leadership of the Soviet Union was shot.[28] The Chinese Communists had a similar objective involving rectification of thought of dissenters. Because of the differing historical traditions of Russia and China, the Chinese proceeded along somewhat divergent lines from those of their Russian *confreres.*

The Chinese Communists attempted to marry the dialectical materialism of Marx, an essentially Western European mode of thinking, with the ancient tenets of Confucianism with its emphasis on rectitude, correct conduct and correct thinking in the service of the state. After their accession to power in 1949 they felt it necessary to reorder the thinking of vast numbers of people who presumably had been living in political and philosophical error. They employed a series of techniques embracing individual and group persuasion. These techniques were then applied to Allied prisoners of war who were captured in Korea.[5, 32-34] The North Koreans themselves carried out some attempts at political indoctrination of prisoners of war but at a very crude level. The Chinese took over the direction of many camps after December 1950 and began a campaign of intensive indoctrination. They utilized such techniques as sleep deprivation and the breaking up of cohesive groups among the prisoners as well as depriving them of their military leaders. Their interrogation techniques employed methods of alternating kindness and cruelty but in every case the interrogators confronted the prisoner continuously with his own wickedness and his stubborn refusal to purge himself of incorrect thoughts. This was applied with varying degree of success to both military and civilian prisoners.

Solitary confinement in a continuously lit cell for months or even years was routine for those deemed particularly important or wicked or both. In every case, the captors eventually obtained some kind of signed confession. At some point during the course of the ordeal, every prisoner became confused, bewildered, exhausted and so completely without social cues that he was completely adrift.[39] He would then accede to virtually any demand, at least with one part of his mind. Naturally, the interrogators were trying to ferret out any hidden resistance, but they did not always do so. Among any group of prisoners there are always active collaborators and others who are active resistors. In Korea, the active collaborators among the Americans were predominantly young, of limited education, and from an impoverished background. They tended to have few internalized values.

Upon release, the prisoners did not seem exultant.[24] They appeared apathetic, weary and constricted just as had the concentration camp inmates.[37] The initial interviews reflected initial apathy but within a few days the pent-up anger began to show itself and the patients became extremely irritable and petulant. After return to the United States, follow-up study showed that, at least in those who underwent the longest ordeal, symptoms of anxiety and depression were still present upon follow-up eight or nine years after release.

American prisoners of the Vietnamese underwent experiences similar in kind to those of prisoners of the Japanese, of the North Koreans, of the Chinese Communists, and, to some degree, of the Nazis.[20] Many were imprisoned for seven or eight years and most suffered long periods of solitary confinement. Sensory isolation was one of the worst stressors and was continued, for some men, for months or years at a time. Torture and political indoctrination were carried out in a manner not dissimilar from that of the North Koreans or the Chinese.

These prisoners have all returned to the United States and to an atmosphere different from the ambience following World War II and the Korean War. Although the war itself was extraordinarily unpopular, the prisoners of war have emerged as its only real heroes. They are receiving much greater acclaim than did their predecessors. It is difficult to know *a priori* whether this publicity and outpouring of applause will be helpful in their rehabilitation or deleterious to their interests. In any case, much more extensive medical and social rehabilitation programs are being provided than was the case in the past. Every medical and psychological finding, both normal and abnormal, on the men is being meticulously recorded. For the first time, former prisoners will each have a definitive medical record to assist in the direction of their future treatment. These encyclopedic data will also provide the best documentation of the future course of any medical disabilities which the men may exhibit as time passes.

Similarly, every possible service will be provided to the families of both the former prisoners of war and the missing in action. Every attempt will be made to prevent the appearance of the kind of psychopathological disability seen in the Canadian families of concentration camp victims. In the future, there will be extensive reports which will serve to document the extent to which these severe stresses of war imprisonment result in adverse psychic and psychopathological consequences.

It is now apparent from follow-up studies of concentration camp victims and the American prisoners of war of the Japanese, North

Koreans and North Vietnamese that permanent psychic and psychophysiological damage can occur to adult human beings if they are subjected to prolonged, malignant and cataclysmic stress.[7] If we had access to medical records from Eastern Europe, no doubt there would be further corroboration of the existence of these phenomena among the millions of individuals who have been incarcerated there for political reasons. Although there are doubtless individual predispositions stemming from the imperfections of child rearing, the universality and uniformity of the postimprisonment syndrome argue strongly for a common etiology, namely, the stress encountered in the prison camp situation.

To recapitulate, virtually all the subjects show evidence of persistent underlying anxiety and most display chronic depression. In addition to these two virtually ubiquitous features, apathy, dependence, helplessness and seclusiveness are common. Still other victims are irritable, quarrelsome, suspicious and hostile. Some of the patients, particularly those who suffered from trauma to the head or from hypovitaminosis, show organic brain syndromes with deficits in memory function, abstract thinking and calculation. Psychosomatic symptoms are also almost universal. Among these fatigue, exhaustion, generalized weakness and gastrointestinal symptoms are common. Sleep is usually disturbed with the patients showing insomnia, frequent awakening and nightmares. In the concentration camp victims and in certain of the former prisoners of war there is a pervasive sense of guilt about having survived when so many died.[17] Ostwald and Bittner[31] have described a subgroup of victims of concentration camps who have developed what the authors call a "synecdoche of success." This style of life is characterized by an apparently successful life adjustment based on highly concentrated and aggressive pursuit of success, hiding extreme depression, anxiety and hostility underneath. These victims are outwardly affluent and prosperous but basically unhappy with marked constriction of pleasure, comfort and tranquillity. The authors feel that this phenomenon can be understood in terms of the patients' continuing to perceive the massive threat to existence under which they had always lived as not merely historical but actually as an ever-present reality.

While in some instances it may be clear that the symptoms which the patient displays are purely the result of psychic stress or in others purely the result of physical factors such as disease, malnutrition and trauma, in most instances it is evident that a combination of these etiologic agents superimposed upon the individual's own preexisting physical and psychic strength or weakness have resulted in the evident KZ syndrome. It is earnestly to be hoped that informed and comprehensive rehabilitative measures can abort the appearance of this syndrome in the newly released prisoners of the Vietnamese war, or if not halt it entirely, at least ameliorate its worst effects. The training which many prisoners received prior to entering the war zone might also have had the effect of preventing some future psychic manifestations such as guilt.[40] The age (most over 30), the relatively high rank (field grade officers), the physical and mental toughness (most were professional aircrew of the regular forces), and the cohesiveness of the bulk of American prisoners of the North Vietnamese argue for a more favorable prognosis than that of the prisoners of past conflicts. The future will confirm or deny the accuracy of this hypothesis.

REFERENCES

1. Abel, T.: The sociology of concentration camps. *Soc Forces, 30*:150, 1951.
2. Adamson, J.D., and Judge, C.M.: Residual disability in Hong Kong prisoners of war. *Can Serv Med J, 12*:837, 1956.
3. Anderson, C.L., Boysen, A.M., Esenten, S., Lamb, G., and Shadish, W.R.: Medical experiences in Communist POW camps in Korea: Experiences and observations of five medical officers who were prisoners of war. *JAMA, 156*:120, 1954.
4. Bettelheim, B.: *The Informed Heart: Autonomy in a Mass Age.* Glencoe, Ill., Free Press, 1960.
5. Biderman, A.D.: Effects of Communist indoctrination attempts: Some comments on an Air Force prisoner of war study. *Soc Prob, 6*:304, 1959.
6. Brill, N.Q.: Neuropsychiatric examinations of military personnel recovered from Japanese prison camps. *Bull US Army Med Dept, 5*:429, 1946.
7. ———, and Beebe, G.W.: A follow-up study of war neuroses. V.A. Medical Monograph, 1956.
8. Chodoff, Paul: Effects of extreme coercive and oppressive forces. In Arieti, S. (Ed.): *American Handbook of Psychiatry.* New York, Basic, 1966, vol. 3, p. 384.

9. ————: The German concentration camp as a psychological stress. *Arch Gen Psychiatr, 22*:78, 1970.

10. ————: Late effects of the concentration camp syndrome. *Arch Gen Psychiatr, 8*:323, 1963.

11. Eitinger, L.: Concentration camp survivors in a postwar world. *Am J Orthopsychiatr, 32*:367, 1962.

12. ————: Pathology of the concentration camp syndrome. *Arch Gen Psychiatr, 5*:371, 1961.

13. ————: Preliminary notes on a study of concentration camp survivors in Norway and Israel. *Ann Psychiatr Related Disciplines, 1*:53, 1963.

14. ————: Rehabilitation of concentration camp survivors following concentration camp trauma. *Psychother Psychosom, 17*:42, 1969.

15. ————: *Concentration Camp Survivors in Norway and Israel.* Oslo, Universitetsforlaget, 1964.

16. Freud, Sigmund: *Beyond the Pleasure Principle.* New York, Bantam, 1959.

17. Grauer, H.: Psychodynamics of the survivor syndrome. *Can Psychiatr Assoc J, 14*:617, 1969.

18. Grinker, Roy R., and Spiegel, John P.: *Men Under Stress.* Philadelphia, Blakiston, 1945.

19. Hafner, H.: Psychological disturbances following prolonged persecution. *Soc Psychiatr, 3*:79, 1968.

20. Halloran, A. V.: Comparison of W.W. II, Korean, and Vietnamese prisoners of war. *Minn Med 53*:919, 1970.

21. Jones, Ernest: *The Life and Work of Sigmund Freud. Vol. 1, The Formative Years and the Great Discoveries.* New York, Basic, 1953.

22. ————: *The Life and Work of Sigmund Freud. Vol. 2, 1901-1919 Years of Maturity.* New York, Basic, 1955.

23. ————: *The Life and Work of Sigmund Freud. Vol. 3, 1919-1939 The Last Phase.* New York, Basic, 1957.

24. Lifton, R.J.: Home by ship: Reaction patterns of American prisoners of war repatriated from North Korea. *Am J Psychiatr, 110*:732, 1954.

25. Meerlo, J.: Persecution trauma and the reconditioning of emotional life: A brief survey. *Am J Psychiatr, 125*:1187, 1969.

26. Morgan, H.J., Wright, I.S., and van Ravenswaay, A.: Health of repatriated prisoners of war from the Far East. *JAMA, 130*:995, 1946.

27. Nefzger, M.D.: Follow-up studies of World War II and Korean War prisoners. I. Study plan and mortality findings. *Am J Epidemiol, 91*:123 ,1970.

28. Nikolai, Ivanovich: *The Great Purge Trial,* 1st ed. Edited with notes by Tucker, Robert C., and Cohen, Stephen S. New York, Grosset and Dunlap, 1965.

29. Nunberg, Herman, and Federn, Ernst: *Minutes of the Vienna Psycho-Analytic Society, Vol. 1, 1906-1908.* New York, International Universities Press, 1962.

30. Nunberg, Herman, and Federn, Ernst: *Minutes of the Vienna Psycho-Analytic Society, Vol. 2, 1908-1911.* New York, International Universities Press, 1967.
31. Ostwald, P., and Bittner, E.: Life adjustment after severe persecution. *Am J Psychiatr, 124*:1393, 1969.
32. Schein, E.H.: Reaction patterns to severe, chronic stress in American Army prisoners of war of the Chinese. *J Soc Issues, 13*:21, 1957.
33. ————: Brainwashing and totalitarianism in modern society. *World Politics, 2*:430, 1959.
34. ————: The Chinese indoctrination program for prisoners of war. *Psychiatry, 19*:149, 1956.
35. Segal, H.A.: Initial psychiatric findings of recently repatriated prisoners of war. *Am J Psychiatr, 111(5)*:358, 1954,
36. Sigal, J.J., and Rakoff, V.: Concentration camp survival. A pilot study of effects on the second generation. *Can Psychiatr Assoc J, 16*:393, 1971.
37. Strassman, H.D., Thaler, M.B., and Schein, E.H.: A prisoner of war syndrome: Apathy as a reaction to severe stress. *Am J Psychiatr, 112*:998, 1956.
38. Strom, A.: Examination of Norwegian ex-concentration camp prisoners. *J Neuropsychiatr, 4*:43, 1962.
39. Walter, R.H., Callagan, J.E., and Newman, A.F.: Effect of solitary confinement on prisoners. *Am J Psychiatr, 119*:771, 1963.
40. West, L.J.: Psychiatric aspects of training for honorable survival as a prisoner of war. *Am J Psychiatr, 115*:329, 1958.
41. Wolf, S., and Ripley, H.S.: Reactions among allied prisoners of war subjected to three years of imprisonment and torture by the Japanese. *Am J Psychiatr, 104*:180, 1947.

≷∧∧∧∧∧∧∧∧∧∧∧∧∧∧∧≷

Chapter XIII

U.S. NAVY UNDERWATER DEMOLITION
TEAM TRAINING:
BIOCHEMICAL STUDIES

ROBERT T. RUBIN AND RICHARD H. RAHE

IT HAS BEEN KNOWN for a number of years, following the pioneering work of Hinkle et al.,[8] that the development of illness in a
population is not distributed homogeneously throughout that population but rather is concentrated in a relatively small "sick" subgroup.
Similarly, the development of multiple illnesses is concentrated in
yet a smaller part of this illness-prone subgroup. Because this phenomenon is of immense practical as well as epidemiological importance, studies were undertaken on U. S. Navy men aboard ship to
define factors in a man's life situation that influence his development
of illness.[6, 7, 16, 17, 21, 25, 22-24]

Factors studied have included ship's activity (combat or port);
the men's work (division) assignment; age, rank, time in service,
education and other demographic variables; and the amount of life
change experienced prior to an overseas cruise as assessed by a standard questionnaire, the Schedule of Recent Experience. These studies are presented in detail elsewhere in this volume. In brief, our
findings replicated those of Hinkle in that illnesses were clustered
in small subgroups of ships' populations, which included those men
who were relatively young, inexperienced, of low rating and in the
service for a short time, and assigned to grueling jobs in the more
hostile environments aboard ship. The men who developed more

illnesses also had higher life change scores computed from the Schedule of Recent Experience.

Large-scale epidemiological studies of patterns of illness onset permit the application of techniques of multivariate analysis—in this instance to determine the relative influence of each of the afore-mentioned factors, but this type of study will not elucidate the psycho-physiologic mechanisms underlying the clinical expression of ill-ness. Toward this end, behavorial-biochemical correlative studies have been conducted to test the responses of biochemical variables in certain stress situations as a way of examining psychosomatic intervening variables.

UNDERWATER DEMOLITION TEAM STUDIES

One program that has lent itself well to this approach is the Navy underwater demolition team (UDT) training program.[14, 15, 18-20, 27-29] This is an arduous four-month-long course that is conducted several times each year. Young, physically healthy, well-motivated enlisted men and officers volunteer for the program, either directly after recruit training or following some years in the Navy. The training schedule includes periods of intense physical stress, intense psycho-logical stress and periods of both.

The first month of training is devoted primarily to physical con-ditioning. Daily distance runs up to six miles are conducted along the beach. Strict military discipline is emphasized, and classroom sessions often are followed by periods of calisthenics. Many of the men have only rudimentary swimming skills, and during this first month distance swims up to a mile in length are begun, first in a heated pool and then in the ocean. In the third week the men re-turn to the pool and the face mask is introduced, which the men later use in their ocean swims.

Physical conditioning peaks during the fifth week of the course, when the men go through "hell week." During this week the daily training schedule is replaced by a twenty-four-hour routine, and it is usual for trainees to get only a few hours of sleep per twenty-four hours. The major objective of the instructors during this week is to prove to the trainees that no matter how tired they feel and how low their morale, it is possible, indeed of vital importance, to keep going. The men have no concept of an end to the exercises they are re-quired to complete. They may be allowed to go to sleep at 2 or

3 AM, only to be awakened five minutes later. Observers of hell week have reported that for the first day or two the trainees display considerable anxiety and feelings of being overwhelmed by the grueling schedule. During the third and fourth days the men develop a "second wind" and are fairly alert with a seemingly good morale. During the last days of this week, however, sheer exhaustion is evidenced in the trainees by greatly prolonged reaction times, distractability, and lack of *esprit de corps*. The attrition rate for the course ranges from 30 to 70 percent. Most of the men drop out by the end of hell week, usually with some subjective physical complaint or an overt illness or injury.

Following hell week there is an easier period of two weeks of classroom exercises, focusing on the care and use of diving and demolition equipment. Then the new equipment is introduced into use, beginning with swim fins and weapons. Day and night ocean swims are conducted as well as helicopter drops and pickups. After the first two months of the course, the class is divided into two groups. One group continues for four weeks with classroom work, the introduction of scuba gear, day and night compass swims, and mine searching, while the other group goes to an offshore island for demolition training. For the last month of the course each group switches to the other program.

The study of the UDT trainees involved the periodic administration of several questionnaires as well as the collection of blood samples. A random sample of the trainees was obtained prior to the start of the course by selecting every third name from an alphabetical roster of a class of about 100 men. The resulting sample of 32 men was then observed throughout the course until they either dropped out or successfully graduated at the end of four months. Fasting blood samples were collected from the subjects at 6 AM three times a week for the first four weeks. During the fifth week (hell week), blood samples were taken on four consecutive days. During the sixth through the eighth weeks of the course, blood samples were taken twice a week. When the group was divided for offshore demolition training, blood samples were taken only from the group remaining behind for scuba training. For the purposes of this report, however, the focus will be on the entire group during the first two months of training.

Behavioral data were obtained both as impressions of the men's emotional states and reactions to training gathered by the medical corpsmen at the time of the blood drawings and by periodic conferences about the men with the class instructors. Each time blood samples were taken the men completed a standardized mood and attitude questionnaire. The aforementioned Schedule of Recent Experience was completed only at the start of the course.

In an attempt to elucidate the effects of the physical and psychological extremes of the training on the physiological functioning of the men, three biochemical measures were chosen for assay in the blood (serum) samples: uric acid, cholesterol and cortisol.[2-5,11] It was hypothesized that changes in each would reflect different aspects of the training program. The rationale for this hypothesis is as follows:

Although it had been generally believed that both serum uric acid and cholesterol were quite stable, except in persons with metabolic diseases such as gout or hypercholesterolemia, studies in the past fifteen years have documented that a wide range of serum levels of both metabolites is displayed in humans, and certain psychological and behavioral variables correlate strongly with elevated uric acid and cholesterol levels.[9,10,19]

Psychological, social and behavioral variables which appear to correlate positively with elevated levels of serum uric acid include relatively stable parameters, such as social class, as well as short-term psychological states, such as motivation. In particular, both transient and long-term elevations in uric acid levels have been noted to accompany achievement-oriented behavior. The person with an elevated serum uric acid level has been described as attacking current situational challenges with zest and confidence. He characteristically performs well and often attains leadership roles.

Certain psychological and behavioral variables appear to correlate positively with elevated serum cholesterol. The particular kinds of psychosocial conflict do not seem to be as important as how the subject interprets and attempts to handle them. Often the individual with elevated serum cholesterol describes himself as being overwhelmed by environmental demands. He appears to be self-critical, adheres to social norms, places a high value on being dependable, and attempts to manage life demands by conscientiousness, perseverance, and time-conscious hurrying.[20]

Although both persons with high serum uric acid levels and persons with high serum cholesterol levels have been described as hardworking and frequently successful, an important distinction is how they perceive their current life situations. Persons with high serum uric acid concentrations appear to consider life demands as enjoyable challenges. Persons with high serum cholesterol concentrations, on the other hand, appear to consider current life stresses as burdens under which they might not bear up, and they tend to react with feelings of aggression, repressed hostility, self-criticism, guilt and depression.

The common psychological variable that correlates most highly with elevated serum cortisol levels is subjectively felt anxiety. There is an extensive literature on the influence of stress situations, both naturally occurring and experimentally contrived, on the activation of the hypothalamic-pituitary-adrenal cortical axis.[12,21] Practically any shift in life situation which evokes an emotional response may activate the adrenal cortex. Pertinent and specific social, psychological and behavioral variables which appear to correlate highly with elevated serum cortisol include introduction into a novel environment, first-time experience of experimental procedures, and anticipation of stress situations as well as the initial encounter with the stress situation itself. Neither perceptual and social isolation nor water immersion with normal subjects has resulted in increased serum cortisol levels aside from the first-time effect, and physical exercise per se appears to cause no change in adrenal cortical activity.

Individual differences in serum cortisol levels have been related to physiologic and anthropometric variables, to sleep-wake patterns and physical illness, and to the psychological variables of felt anxiety, absence of denial, awareness of threat of injury or loss, and failing ego defenses.[12,26,27] In general, the more pronounced any of these latter psychological variables is, the greater is the concomitant activation of the pituitary-adrenal cortical axis. For an individual at any given time, it appears that the psychological determinant of the level of adrenal cortical activity is the interaction between internal ego defense strength and stressful external milieu circumstances; this interaction has been noted in military men under combat conditions.[1]

Results

Twenty of the thirty-two originally selected trainees completed the UDT program. The percentage of dropouts in the sample (37%) was close to the overall percentage of drops from the entire class (31%). During the first two or three weeks of training, serum uric acid levels were lower, cholesterol levels were higher, and cortisol levels were lower for the twelve men who dropped out of training than were the values for the twenty men who completed the course. These mean differences, however, were not statistically significant.

On the mood and attitude questionnaire given each time blood was sampled, the men who withdrew from the program registered more complaints about the program and indicated more psychophysiologic symptoms than did the men who completed the course. On the Schedule of Recent Experience, the men who withdrew from UDT training for primarily medical reasons registered a greater mean number of life change units for the year prior to training than did the men who completed the course. These mean differences were statistically significant (p < 0.01).[15]

Biochemical differences between the men who withdrew and the men who finished UDT training suggested that the unsuccessful group was more complaining and less motivated (lower uric acid) and was more concerned with somatic symptoms and more threatened by failure (higher cholesterol). The behavioral data and the biochemical data, except for cortisol, were consistent in their interrelationships. It would have been expected that the group who voluntarily dropped from the training would have responded with more anxiety as reflected by higher cortisol level, but this was not the case. Voluntary dropouts did register significantly elevated subjective anxiety on the Cornell Medical Index Health Questionnaire, however, compared to successful candidates.[15] Between January 6 and January 20, the first two weeks of training, physical conditioning and progressive distance swims, first in the swimming pool and then in the ocean, were taking place. Uric acid levels fell and cholesterol levels rose during this time. The first-day mean uric acid level of 7.78 mg/100 ml was remarkable in that it was in the hyperuricemic range, perhaps reflecting the subjects' general enthusiasm and high levels of motivation at the start of the course. Cortisol values during these first two weeks were high, averaging 22 µg/100 ml, and were clearly in the "stress" range for 6 AM samples.[21] A peak in cortisol occurred coincident with the start of swimming practice (January 9); most of the men were better runners than swimmers during the early part of the course. Over the next two weeks mean cortisol values declined as the men became accustomed to the swimming tasks.

On January 23 the men returned to the heated pool and were given face masks. Uric acid levels continued to decline up to this point, and cholesterol levels conversely continued to rise, both following the same trend from the beginning of the course. On this day, however, a statistically significant increase in cortisol occurred, apparently related to the use of the face mask. Most of the trainees had little prior underwater diving experience, and the introduction of technical gear was met with overt anxiety by many trainees. Over the next few days long ocean swims with the face mask were practiced. Uric acid levels remained low, and both cholesterol and cortisol levels declined somewhat.

January 30 marked the first day of hell week. The men's attitudes and behavior changed dramatically during this week. On the first day they saw the week as an enormous hurdle they had to surmount, and they struggled to accomplish this end. By the second day the men generally realized they could not possibly continue such a pace, and they began to conserve their energies. By the end of the week their tolerance for the grueling schedule had been depleted. On the first day of hell week mean serum uric acid concentration was relatively low while cholesterol had significantly risen to a relatively high level. By the next day uric acid had risen significantly, only to fall once more toward the end of the week. Serum cholesterol concentration similarly demonstrated a significant fall during the latter part of the week. Mean serum cortisol peaked significantly on the first day, remained elevated on the second day, fell significantly on the third day, and again peaked significantly on the fourth day. Cortisol values reached their highest levels of the entire course during this week. The wide fluctuation in day-to-day values for all three measures was most likely related to the schedule of this week, which included sleep deprivation and altered sleep-wake cycles as well as severe physical exertion.

During the following sixth week (February 7 to February 14) the men had a relatively easy schedule. During this week serum uric acid was at its lowest mean concentration. The men also began classroom reconnaissance work at this time, and many of the trainees found it to be quite difficult. Serum cholesterol concentration rose significantly during this week. On February 16, during the seventh week, swim fins and UDT weaponry were introduced. Besides having inherent anxiety concerning the handling of weapons, many of the relatively good swimmers, as well as most of the poor ones, had difficulty in learning to swim with diving fins. Uric acid levels increased significantly during this time of return to active work in the field, but cholesterol also increased significantly to the highest level of the entire first two months of training. A significant increase in serum cortisol also occurred on this day of exposure to new equipment and techniques, but mean cortisol values declined over the next week as ocean swimming with fins was practiced.

On February 23 the men experienced their first helicopter drops and pickups. Uric acid levels were down, and cholesterol values remained high. There again was an increase in serum cortisol on this day, which declined over the next week of helicopter maneuvers. At the end of the first two months the men were divided into two groups, as mentioned earlier. Uric acid levels rose sharply, perhaps reflecting a feeling of success with the first half of the course and a renewed sense of motivation and challenge concerning the second half. Cholesterol and cortisol both declined toward the end of the first two months, which followed lessened feelings of anxiety and being overburdened as this phase of the program drew to a close.

During the month of diving training the behavioral and biochemical changes followed much the same pattern of interrelatedness as they did during the first two months. These data have been presented previously.[15,24] The changes in mean serum levels for the first two months of the course suffice to illustrate group trends.

Although the group of twenty men was homogeneous with respect to age, sex, health status and probable lack of genetic predisposition to hyperuricemia or hypercholesterolemia, there were statistically significant differences between subjects in individual mean level of uric acid, cholesterol and cortisol.[28] Each subject had a fairly restricted variability of all three biochemical measures compared to the

Life Stress and Illness

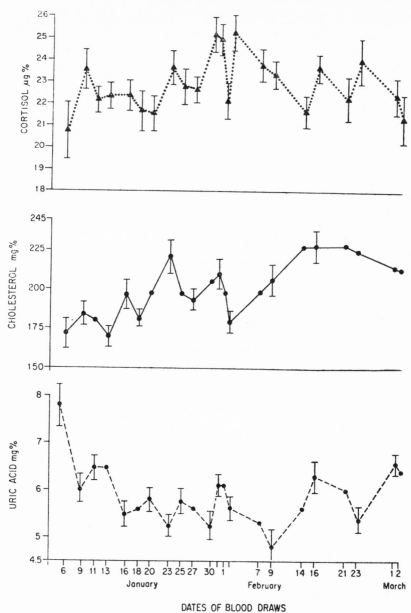

Figure XIII-1. Mean serum uric acid, cholesterol and cortisol levels during UDT training.

differences in these measures between subjects (Table XIII-I), in spite of the considerable changes in life situations for all the subjects simultaneously as the training program unfolded. The individual means of serum uric acid levels ranged between 4.55 and 7.08 mg/100 ml, and individual variabilities were 9 to 18 percent of the individual mean values. None of the subjects was statistically hyperuricemic (greater than 7.00 mg/100 ml), with the possible exception of subject 11, whose serum uric acid levels were quite variable. The individual means of serum cholesterol levels ranged between 173 and 244 mg/100 ml, and individual variabilities were 8 to 20 percent of the individual means. None of the subjects appeared to be consistently hypercholesterolemic. The individual means of serum cortisol levels ranged between 19.8 and 25.9 µg/100 ml, and individual variabilities were 10 to 25 percent of the individual means. These mean levels were comparable to those found in normal subjects undergoing a variety of fairly intense, naturally occurring stressful experiences.

TABLE XIII-I. INDIVIDUAL MEANS AND STANDARD DEVIATIONS
FOR SERUM URIC ACID, CHOLESTEROL AND CORTISOL

Subject No.	Uric Acid (mg/100 ml)	Cholesterol (mg/100 ml)	Cortisol (µg/100 ml)
1	5.69 ± 1.05	212 ± 29	23.8 ± 5.9
2	5.40 ± 0.79	178 ± 36	22.1 ± 2.5
3	6.14 ± 1.10	215 ± 24	20.5 ± 2.8
4	5.73 ± 0.54	219 ± 21	23.3 ± 2.3
5	5.87 ± 0.80	183 ± 36	23.1 ± 2.9
6	4.55 ± 0.57	203 ± 25	20.3 ± 3.7
7	6.25 ± 0.66	181 ± 20	21.9 ± 2.8
8	5.97 ± 0.88	183 ± 28	23.7 ± 3.0
9	5.47 ± 1.00	179 ± 36	20.9 ± 2.9
10	6.25 ± 0.92	242 ± 26	23.1 ± 3.2
11	7.08 ± 1.08	229 ± 32	23.9 ± 3.7
12	6.79 ± 1.13	180 ± 24	19.8 ± 3.0
13	5.07 ± 0.76	214 ± 29	23.8 ± 3.0
14	6.08 ± 0.77	215 ± 24	25.9 ± 4.1
15	5.00 ± 0.66	213 ± 18	21.8 ± 3.6
16	6.66 ± 1.07	178 ± 31	23.3 ± 3.5
17	5.96 ± 0.78	173 ± 29	22.4 ± 3.1
18	6.30 ± 0.85	223 ± 21	23.3 ± 3.5
19	5.52 ± 0.96	244 ± 35	21.7 ± 3.4
20	6.17 ± 0.99	224 ± 33	20.7 ± 4.1

The average intersubject correlations[13] among the three biochemical variables were all of low order (Table XIII-II), suggesting that in our subjects these measures bore little relationship to each other. Furthermore, the intraindividual correlations among these variables showed a considerable range of values. These data indicate that a cross-sectional statistical analysis of intercorrelations among serum uric acid, cholesterol and cortisol levels can mask the considerable variations found in longitudinal, intraindividual correlations among these measures. The data further indicate that even in a homogenous group of normal subjects in the same stressful environment there may be a marked individuality in patterns of biochemical response and adaptation. This individuality is exemplified by the following four illustrations of individual subjects' uric acid, cholesterol and cortisol patterns along with notations of seemingly key concomitant physi-

TABLE XIII-II. INTERCORRELATIONS OF SERUM URIC ACID,
CHOLESTEROL AND CORTISOL FOR EACH SUBJECT

Subject No.	Uric Acid: Cholesterol	Uric Acid: Cortisol	Cholesterol: Cortisol
(Average)	(− 0.01)	(+ 0.18)	(+ 0.19)
1	+ 0.05	+ 0.01	+ 0.11
2	+ 0.15	+ 0.30	+ 0.07
3	− 0.24	− 0.08	− 0.09
4	− 0.04	+ 0.12	+ 0.16
5	− 0.37	− 0.12	− 0.20
6	+ 0.27	− 0.10	− 0.35
7	+ 0.16	− 0.22	+ 0.22
8	+ 0.13	+ 0.04	+ 0.05
9	+ 0.41	− 0.06	− 0.10
10	− 0.37	+ 0.08	− 0.28
11	− 0.41	− 0.24	+ 0.46
12	− 0.32	+ 0.12	+ 0.17
13	− 0.28	+ 0.02	− 0.27
14	− 0.20	+ 0.21	+ 0.19
15	− 0.29	− 0.29	+ 0.20
16	+ 0.16	+ 0.22	+ 0.45
17	− 0.14	− 0.32	+ 0.10
18	+ 0.15	0.00	+ 0.07
19	− 0.12	− 0.07	+ 0.14
20	− 0.28	− 0.27	+ 0.03

cal and psychological factors. All four subjects completed the course.

Figure XIII-2 represents a trainee who was described by his instructors as having a very good attitude throughout his training. His serum uric acid and cholesterol curves were prototypic of those men described by the instructors as desirable UDT candidates. Especially characteristic of the good candidate, as seen in this subject, was the initial elevated serum uric acid (8 to 9 mg/100 ml) along with a low serum cholesterol concentration. Initial cortisol levels, although in the "stress" range,[26] were lower than those of most of the other subjects. Throughout hell week (January 30 to February 5) and the subsequent classroom portion of training, his performance was above average, and his concomitant uric acid levels remained relatively high. The increase in his cholesterol values during the first weeks of the course was modal (Fig. XIII-1), and cortisol levels did not fluctuate widely during hell week. Both cholesterol and cortisol peaked on February 16, the day of the introduction of swim fins and weaponry, but they declined markedly over the next month as he progressed into diving training. A substantial peak of uric acid occurred on March 23, the day his group began mine searching and long compass swims. Cortisol also peaked sharply on that day. This subject's lack of difficulty with diving training was paralleled by consistently low serum cholesterol values.

Figure XIII-3 represents a man who typified the few who were

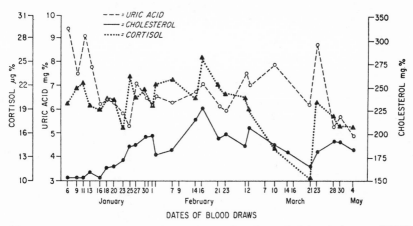

Figure XIII-2. Serum uric acid, cholesterol and cortisol levels in one UDT trainee.

marginally suited for UDT training. According to his instructors he tried to slide by with a minimum of effort. He demonstrated no initial elevation of serum uric acid. Over the entire training period the only peak in this man's uric acid concentration came at a time when he was highly aroused about his automobile having been impounded at the amphibious base (January 23). He had little difficulty with the course material until diving training. Here he revealed a rapidly rising serum cortisol level and a prominent peak of cholesterol coincident with his final examination compass swims (April 25). Followup information on this trainee revealed that after graduation he continued to have difficulties in diving and remained a borderline frogman in terms of his overall proficiency.

Figure XIII-4 presents data on a trainee who began the course with what was described by his instructors as "poor motivation." This subject failed to show a high initial serum uric acid concentration, but he did have high initial cortisol levels. He had a rapid rise in serum cholesterol level when he began distance swimming during the first two weeks of the course. His cholesterol concentration peaked during hell week (January 31) and then climbed to nearly 300 mg/100 ml during his borderline classroom work and distance swims with newly acquired diving fins (February 21). Cortisol levels also were high at this time, and uric acid levels remained quite low. Since this subject was in the second group, he took his demolition training prior to diving instruction (as did the preceding subject). When diving

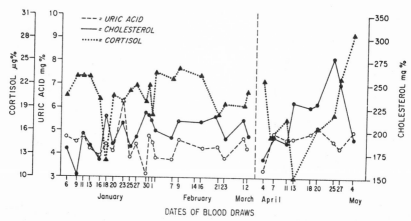

Figure XIII-3. Serum uric acid, cholesterol and cortisol levels in a second UDT trainee.

training began, his instructors noted that his attitude had improved markedly. He was very attentive toward the course materials and tried hard to overcome his poor swimming abilities. A high peak in his serum uric acid was seen at this time (April 7). He continued, however, to have difficulties with his swimming, and at the time of his first compass swim (April 11) he demonstrated another large peak in serum cholesterol. Cortisol levels continued to be elevated during this time. During diving training his uric acid concentration quickly dropped and during the final examination compass swims (April 27) he developed his highest cholesterol concentration. He failed his first diving exam.

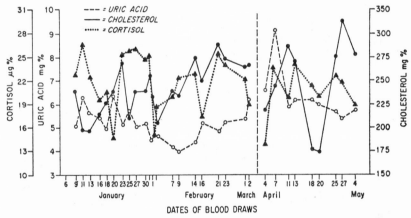

Figure XIII-4. Serum uric acid, cholesterol and cortisol levels in a third UDT trainee.

Figure XIII-5 represents a subject who was noted by his instructors to have been a highly attentive trainee from the start of the course. He began the program with a dramatic elevation in serum uric acid concentration (10 mg/100 ml). However, he was a below-average swimmer, and the first peaks in his serum cholesterol concentration occurred at the beginning of distance and ocean swimming (January 11 and 16). His cholesterol then returned to a very low level until another peak occurred at the introduction of diving fins and UDT weaponry (February 16). Both uric acid and cortisol also increased prominently at this time. The subject, obviously a weak swimmer, had great difficulty with his fins but was noted to try hard despite his limitations. Cortisol peaked on the day of his first compass swims (March 14). His excellent attitude persisted, and he progressed satisfactorily through diving training. This progress was accompanied by relatively elevated serum uric acid levels and very low serum cholesterol concentrations, as well as decreasing cortisol values.

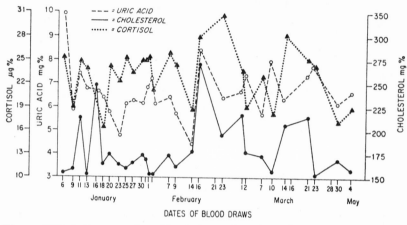

Figure XIII-5. Serum uric acid, cholesterol and cortisol levels in a fourth UDT trainee.

Summary and Discussion

The biochemical data presented above, when considered together with the day-to-day program of the course, suggest that elevations in mean serum uric acid levels occurred coincidentally with eagerly accepted tasks at a time of strong motivation (beginning and first two week of course), with the introduction of new and challenging techniques, and with the preparation for subsequent long-term grueling tasks, such as hell week. Uric acid levels were initially high, declined for the first month, and then gradually rose toward the end of the second month. Individual trainees demonstrated substantial peaks in their serum uric acid levels when they were noted to be alert, attentive and eager for training. The twelve men who withdrew from training had a lower mean uric acid level at the beginning of training than did the ultimately successful trainees.

Elevations in mean serum cholesterol levels occurred in situations evocative of anxiety and fear of failure (first ocean swim, introduction of face mask, start of hell week, and introduction of fins and weapons) and during periods of relatively little physical exercise (two weeks of classroom work). Individuals who had marked difficulties with their swimming and who initially failed their final examination compass swims demonstrated large concomitant elevations in their serum cholesterol levels. The trainees who withdrew from the course tended to have higher initial cholesterol levels than those who graduated.

Elevations in mean serum cortisol levels occurred coincidentally with novel experiences about which the men had some anticipatory anxiety. The introduction of new equipment (face mask, fins and weapons) was consistently met with increased adrenal cortical activity. This anxiety surrounding new equipment apparently was not obviated by a return to more comfortable surroundings, for example, the introduction of the face mask in the heated pool following a week of long ocean swims. Also, new tasks that were anticipated as being difficult (initial distance swims, hell week, helicopter drops and pickups) generally resulted in increased adrenal cortical activity. However, as each new technique was practiced and became familiar to the trainees (progressive distance swims, ocean swims with the face mask and diving fins, helicopter drops and pickups) cortisol levels declined, even though increasing demands for the use of the new technique were being made by the instructors. The determinant of transient increases in adrenal cortical activity therefore seemed to be the anticipation of an unknown situation more than the inherent difficulty or stress of the situation itself, and a rapid adaptation to the actual stress appeared to occur during each new phase. The transient anticipatory increases in serum cortisol occurred against a background of fairly high sustained levels of adrenal cortical activity throughout the entire course.

These cortisol levels were comparable to the serum cortisol concentrations found in subjects undergoing a variety of fairly intense, naturally occurring stressful experiences, including the stress of major physical injury, indicating that UDT training is a chronically anxiety-provoking experience of considerable magnitude. Although the threat of physical injury or death is minimal, failure to complete the course results in a considerable loss of peer group respect. There are only two possible alternatives for handling stress: press on regardless, or drop out. The chronically elevated mean serum cortisol levels appear to be related to these unique aspects of the course.

It is apparent, then, that the changes in each biochemical variable studied—uric acid, cholesterol and cortisol—could be logically related to the various day-to-day requirements and challenges of the UDT programs as spelled out in the activity schedule and as learned from the UDT instructors. This relationship was discernible both for the class as a whole (mean changes) and for individual trainees, as exemplified above. Uric acid did appear to be increased during times of high motivation and confidence in the trainees, cholesterol appeared to be elevated when the men felt overburdened and close to the limits of their tolerance as well as when they were physically less active, and elevated cortisol levels appeared to reflect the continuing global stresses of the course as well as the anticipation of intense but transient stress periods superimposed on the ongoing training activities, which were novel and potentially threatening.

REFERENCES

1. Bourne, P.G.: Urinary 17-OHCS levels in two combat situations. In Bourne, P.G. (Ed.): *The Psychology and Physiology of Stress: With Reference to Special Studies of the Vietnam War.* New York, Academic Press, 1969, p. 95.
2. Clark, B.R., and Rubin, R.T.: New fluorometric method for the determination of cortisol in serum. *Anal Biochem, 29*:31, 1969.
3. ———, Rubin, R.T., and Arthur, R.J.: A new micro-method for the determination of cholesterol in serum. *Anal Biochem, 24*:27, 1968.
4. ———, Rubin, R.T., Kales, A., and Poland, R.: Comparison of fluorometric method for urinary cortisol with modified Portersilber method for 17-OHCS. *Clin Chim Acta, 27*:364, 1970.
5. ———, Rubin, R.T., and Poland, R.E.: Modification of new fluorometric method for serum and urine cortisol. *Biochem Med, 5*:177, 1971.
6. Doll, R.E.; Rubin, R.T., and Gunderson, E.K.E.: Life stress and illness patterns in the U.S. Navy II. Demographic variables and illness onset in an attack carrier's crew. *Arch Environ Health, 19*:748, 1969.
7. Gunderson, E.K.E., Rahe, R.H., and Arthur, R.J.: The epidemiology of illness in naval environments II. Demographic, social background, and occupational factors. *Milit Med, 135*:453, 1970.
8. Hinkle, L.E., Pinsky, R.H., Bross, I.D.J., and Plummer, N.: The distribution of sickness disability in a homogeneous group of "healthy adult men." *Am J Hygiene, 64*:220, 1956.
9. Jenkins, C.D., Hames, C.G., Zyzanski, S.J., Rosenman, R., and Friedman, M.: Psychological traits and serum lipids. *Psychosom Med, 31*:115, 1969.
10. Katz, J.L., and Weiner, H.: Psychosomatic considerations in hyperuricemia and gout. *Psychosom Med, 34*:165, 1972.

11. Liddle, L., Seegmiller, J.E., and Laster, L.: The enzymatic spectro-photometric method for determination of uric acid. *J Lab Clin Med, 54*:903, 1959.

12. Mason, J.W.: A review of psychoendocrine research on the pituitary-adrenal cortical system. *Psychosom Med, 30*:576, 1968.

13. McNemar, Q.: *Psychological Statistics,* 4th ed. New York, John Wiley and Sons, 1969, p. 158.

14. Rahe, R.H., and Arthur, R.J.: Stressful underwater demolition training: Serum urate and cholesterol variability. *JAMA, 202*: 1052, 1967.

15. ————, Biersner, R., Ryman, D., and Arthur, R.J.: Psychosocial predictors of illness behavior and failure in stressful training. *J Health Soc Behav,* in press.

16. ————, Gunderson, E.K.E., and Arthur, R.J.: Demographic and psychosocial factors in acute illness reporting. *J Chronic Dis, 23*:245, 1970.

17. ————, Mahan, J.L., Arthur, R.J., and Gunderson, E.K.E.: The epidemiology of illness in naval environments I. Illness types, distribution, severities, and relationship to life change. *Milit Med, 135*:443, 1970.

18. ————, Rubin, R.T., Arthur, R.J., and Clark, B.R.: Serum uric acid and cholesterol variability: A comprehensive view of underwater demolition team training. *JAMA, 206*:2875, 1968.

19. ————, Rubin, R.T., and Gunderson, E.K.E.: Measures of subjects' motivation and affect correlated with their serum uric acid, cholesterol, and cortisol. *Arch Gen Psychiatr, 26*:357, 1972.

20. ————, Rubin, R.T., Gunderson, E.K.E., and Arthur, R.J.: Psychologic correlates of serum cholestrol in man: A longitudinal study. *Psychosom Med, 33*:399, 1971.

21. Rubin, R.T., Gunderson, E.K.E., and Arthur, R.J.: Life stress and illness patterns in the U.S. Navy III. Prior life change and illness onset in an attack carrier's crew. *Arch Environ Health, 19*:753, 1969.

22. ————, Gunderson, E.K.E., and Arthur, R.J.: Life stress and illness patterns in the U.S. Navy V. Prior life change and illness onset in a battleship's crew. *J Psychosom Res, 15*:89, 1971.

23. ————, Gunderson, E.K.E., and Arthur, R.J.: Life stress and illness patterns in the U.S. Navy IV. Environmental and demographic variables in relation to illness onset in a battleship's crew. *J Psychosom Res, 15*:277, 1971.

24. ————, Gunderson, E.K.E., and Arthur, R.J.: Life stress and illness patterns in the U.S. Navy VI. Environmental, demographic, and prior life change variables in relation to illness onset in naval aviators during a combat cruise. *Psychosom Med, 34*:533, 1972.

25. ————, Gunderson, E.K.E., and Doll, R.E.: Life stress and illness patterns in the U.S. Navy I. Environmental variables and illness onset in an attack carrier's crew. *Arch Environ Health, 19*:740, 1969.

26. ————, and Mandell, A.J.: Adrenal cortical activity in pathological emotional states: A review. *Am J Psychiatr, 123*:387, 1966.

27. ————, Rahe, R.H., Arthur, R.J., and Clark, B.R.: Adrenal cortical activity changes during underwater demolition team training. *Psychosom Med, 31*:553, 1969.

28. ————, Rahe, R.H., Clark, B.R., and Arthur, R.J.: Serum uric acid, cholesterol, and cortisol levels: Inter-relationships in normal men under stress. *Arch Intern Med, 125*:815, 1970.

29. ————, Rahe, R.H., Gunderson, E.K.E., and Clark, B.R.: Motivation and serum uric acid levels. *Percept Mot Skills, 30*:794, 1970.

Chapter XIV

BIOCHEMICAL AND NEUROENDOCRINE RESPONSES TO SEVERE PSYCHOLOGICAL STRESS:

1. U.S. Navy Aviator Study
2. Some General Observations

ROBERT T. RUBIN*

1. U.S. NAVY AVIATOR STUDY

AN EXTRAORDINARY stress circumstance in the U.S. Navy in which behavioral and biochemical correlates were studied was that of student aviators making their first aircraft carrier landings in the F-4B Phantom jet aircraft.[25, 31, 32] In contrast to the UDT experience, landing on an aircraft carrier is a complex technical task that requires considerable prior training and is an extremely hazardous undertaking during the last few seconds of flight. A number of perceptual-motor factors are involved in flying, which include precision control, spatial orientation, multilimb coordination, response orientation, rate control and kinesthetic discrimination. The complexity of adequate aircraft handling is further increased by the requirement of touching down on a carrier deck that is angled with respect to the direction of movement of the ship and that is pitching, rolling and yawing. The training program approaches carrier landings with a graded series of stresses. Night mirror landing practice at the naval air station teaches precision aircraft touchdown on a stable "deck" with little inherent risk. Actual carrier landings are practiced first during the day, then

*The author is currently a recipient of N.I.M.H. Research Scientist Development Award K01-MH47363 and supported by ONR Contract N00014-67-A-0385-0016.

at night. Night carrier landings are much more difficult, as indicated by both objective flight parameters and a 4:1 night:day accident ratio. On a dark, moonless night there is no visible horizon, and the pilot must rely solely on the ship's landing lights for reference.

Both day and night, the pilot must fly the last mile of final approach visually, without an automatic landing system. At one mile from touchdown the entire aircraft carrier appears the size of a pencil eraser held at arm's length. In the particular aircraft flown in this study (F-4B), this last mile is covered in thirty-six seconds. An improper approach may result in (1) a "waveoff" by the landing signal officer who flashes lights signaling the pilot to apply power and abort the landing attempt, (2) a "bolter"—failure of the tail hook to engage the arresting cables which necessitates flying off the end of the flight deck, or (3) a "ramp strike"—hitting the stern of the ship with consequent damage to the aircraft and crew. If the aircraft plunges into the ocean during any phase of the landing attempt, there is essentially no chance of survival. Failure to complete a successful landing after several attempts requires the pilot's returning to the naval air station to land before he runs out of fuel.

The F-4B Phantom jet fighter-bomber is a two-man aircraft. The pilot in the front cockpit, has complete flight control. The radar intercept officer (RIO), in the rear cockpit, monitors the radar and other instruments but has no flight control. He does have excellent visibility. In an emergency both the pilot and the RIO can eject themselves from the aircraft, a procedure not without hazard. The RIO is aware of these hazards and the aircraft's position during the landing attempt, but he must rely completely on the pilot's skill for his own personal safety.

These factors make this training situation quite different from UDT training in terms of the role requirements and responsibilities assigned to the participants. The pairing of active and passive subjects is quite similar to an experimental paradigm in which pairs of monkeys were exposed to a noxious stimulus in an avoidance situation.[6] The "executive" member of the pair (the monkey permitted to press a lever to avoid the noxious stimulus to both) developed gastrointestinal ulcerations, whereas the other monkey, which had no control over the stimulus, did not. The only prior report of human subjects in this type of yoked avoidance paradigm was pairs of men who were exposed to a strong auditory stimulus, one of whom could press a button to avoid a stimulus to both.[11] Again, the "executive" members of the pairs showed a significantly greater amplitude of gastric contractions than did the passive members of the pairs.

Methods

The aviators studied were three successive classes in an advanced military flight training program. The pilots had been in training for two years, and they ranged in age from twenty-two to thirty-two years. The RIO's had been in training for eighteen months and had the same age range as the pilots. All had at least three years of college education, and all were in excellent health during the time of the study.

Psychologic assessments and blood and urine collections were done on these subjects on a nonflying control day and immediately upon their exiting the aircraft after performing the following tasks, in chronological order: night mirror landing practice (MLP) at the naval air station (simulated carrier flight deck), daytime carrier qualifications (DAYQUALS), and nighttime carrier qualifications (NITEQUALS). During each flying period, the pilot made repeated approaches to the ship until he either completed six arrested landings or ran low on fuel, at which time he was sent to a shore landing field. The number of subjects studied varied during each of these phases of training because of last-minute changes in flying schedules and the logistic difficulties inherent in having research personnel stationed aboard the aircraft carrier and at all the possible landing fields in California.

Psychologic data were obtained as follows: First, from the Minnesota Multiphasic Personality Inventory (MMPI), 109 questions comprising the Taylor manifest anxiety scale,[35] the Barron ego strength scale,[3] and the standard K (defensiveness) scale were administered once at the beginning of the study. Eighteen pilots and twenty-one RIO's completed these questions. Ego strength and defensiveness scores were the same for both groups. The RIO's mean score on the manifest anxiety scale was 31 percent higher than the pilots' mean score; however this was not a statistically significant difference. Second, the fear scale of the mood and attitude questionnaire used in the UDT study was administered before each flying period. The pilots' mean score was higher during NITEQUALS than DAYQUALS, and the RIO's mean score was higher than that of the pilots for both of these flying periods. Again, these differences were not statistically significant. Finally, a modified version of the Health Opinion Survey,[15] designed to elicit somatic complaints, was administered before each flying period. On the control day and all three flying days the RIO's reported a greater mean number of somatic complaints than did the pilots; the difference was statistically significant for the control day and for NITEQUALS.

The biochemical variables studied were plasma and urine cortisol,[7-9] as an index of subjective anxiety, and urine 3-methoxy-4-hydroxyphenyl-glycol (MHPG), as an index of brain catecholamine metabolism. MHPG is a neutral metabolite of epinephrine and norepinephrine (NE). About 25 percent of total urine MHPG previously was thought to be derived from the metabolism of brain NE.[32] However, recent correlations in monkeys of decrease in urine MHPG with the depletion of brain NE caused by 6-hydroxydopamine suggest that in primates up to 50 percent of urine MHPG may be derived from brain NE.[20] Because animal studies have demonstrated directly that there is an increased turnover of brain NE under several experimental stress conditions, urine MHPG was measured in the aviators as a possible reflection of changes in brain NE metabolism under the conditions of heightened arousal and concentration occasioned by the carrier landings.

Results

Figure XIV-1 indicates the mean serum cortisol responses for the pilots and RIO's on the control day and for each of the flying periods. The probability levels represent comparisons of the control values to the values for each of the flying periods. With reference to serum cortisol, the mean level of the pilots following all three flying periods was significantly higher than the control mean; a 229 percent increase over control followed the DAYQUALS. In contrast to the pilots, the mean cortisol level of the RIO's was not significantly increased following any flying period compared to the nonflying day; only a 40 percent increase over control followed the DAYQUALS. Although the RIO's evidenced a higher mean cortisol level than the pilots on the control day, the pilots had a higher mean serum level than the RIO's following all three flying periods. The urinary

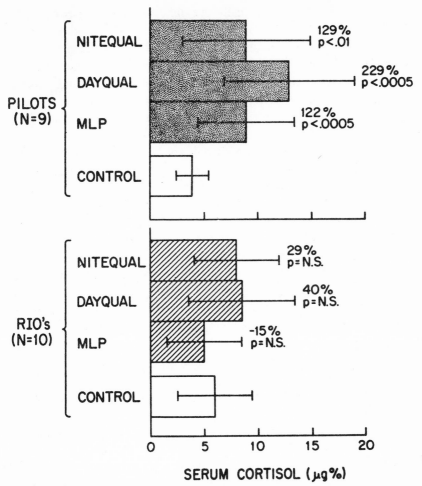

Figure XIV-1. Mean serum cortisol levels in naval aviators.

excretion of cortisol and 17-hydroxycorticosteroid metabolites paralleled the above changes in serum cortisol levels.

These results indicate that aircraft carrier landing practice was considerably more stressful for the pilots than for their RIO's. In the context of the "executive" monkey paradigm, the "executive" naval aviator, who had to perform a highly complex task while avoiding serious potential harm to himself, his partner and his aircraft, showed an unequivocal adrenal cortical stress response. The passive partner, on the other hand, although completely aware of the risks involved, showed only a slight, statistically insignificant adrenal response. This occurred in spite of the fact that the psychological testing demonstrated higher general anxiety levels in the RIO's on all days tested, even though their responsibility was minimal. These findings support the previous work on paired animal and human subjects and point to the importance of assigned role, responsibility and active involvement as factors dominant over more basic personality aspects in the hierarchy of control of adrenal cortical responses. This role difference has been noted in other studies of military populations, in which officers and commanders, who were in decision-making positions and were responsible for the safety and welfare of the men under their command, had higher adrenal responses than did their men.[4]

As with the UDT trainees, some modifying effects of experience and training were suggested by the cortisol responses in the naval aviators. In spite of the greater hazards of night carrier landings, both the pilots and the RIO's showed a somewhat lower adrenal activation during NITEQUALS compared to DAYQUALS, suggesting that some of the novelty of landing a high performance jet on a carrier may have been dissipated following the experience of the day landings. The modifying effects of experience also have been noted in other psychoendocrine studies of military populations.[4, 33, 34]

With reference to urine MHPG, as shown in Figure XIV-2, both groups of aviators (pilots and RIO's) showed statistically significant increases in mean MHPG excretion levels commensurate with the graded series of tasks in the training program. These increases were similar in magnitude for both groups of subjects. If urine MHPG excretion is indeed a reasonably accurate reflection of brain NE metabolism, then the changes in mean MHPG levels would suggest an accelerated turnover of brain NE under the conditions of heightened arousal and alertness during the flying periods compared to the control day. The similar MHPG changes in the pilots and the RIO's imply similar degrees of arousal for each of the flying tasks in these two groups of aviators, with the exception of a greater increase in MHPG excretion for the pilots during NITEQUALS. As outlined above, NITEQUALS was the most hazardous part of the training program, and it is reasonable that the pilots as a group would have manifested a greater degree of arousal and intense concentration than the RIO's during this time.

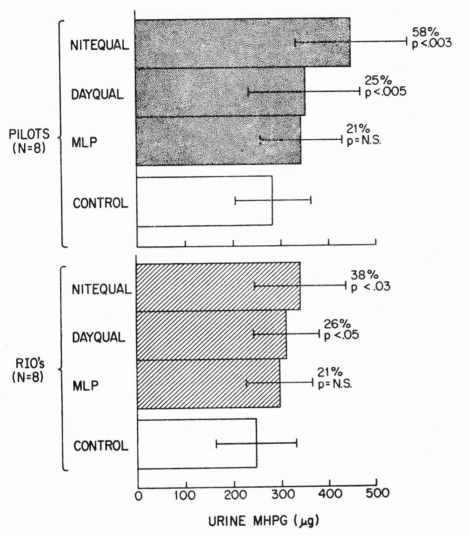

Figure XIV-2. Mean urine MHPG excretion in naval aviators.

Comment

It is of interest to contrast the MHPG excretion data with the serum and urine cortisol data. It was pointed out that the pilots had significant increases in serum cortisol on all three flying days compared to the control day, whereas the RIO's did not. The urine corticosteroid excretion data supported this finding of a greater adrenal cortical stress response in the pilots compared to the RIO's. Although a greater adrenal stress response was expected for NITE-QUALS compared to DAYQUALS, because of the flight factors discussed earlier, serum levels and urine excretion of corticosteroids for both groups of aviators were somewhat lower following the NITEQUAL period. As mentioned above, this finding suggested that some psychoendocrine adaptation to the stress of carrier landings might have occurred between the day and the night periods.

Changes in MHPG excretion, on the other hand, were similar for both the pilots and the RIO's and were commensurate with the difficulty of the tasks. These findings suggest that the corticosteroid and MHPG patterns reflected different aspects of the stress situation. The serum and urine cortisol changes appeared to be related to the anticipatory anxiety attendant to the novelty of a new task. The MHPG changes appeared to be related to the intensity of the concentration, attention and alertness required to perform the task, and these factors did not diminish with experience.

This study of naval aviators attempting their first day and night aircraft carrier landings helps to elucidate the psychophysiology of (1) highly trained pilots required to perform an extremely complex psychomotor task that exposes them to a high degree of physical danger for a short period of time (less than one minute), and (2) equally highly trained radar intercept officers who are passive partners in the same endeavor as the pilots. This set of stressful circumstances, then, is quite different from that of the UDT training program, in which naive subjects are exposed to a relatively nonspecific series of new experiences and challenges, both physical and psychological, over an extended period of time. Two different dimensions of biochemical and neuroendocrine responses were investigated in the aviator study—the influence of role (active vs. passive) on the adrenal cortical stress response, and the effect of heightened arousal and vigilance during a complex task on an indirect measure of brain norepinephrine metabolism.

2. GENERAL NEUROENDOCRINOLOGIC COMMENTS

The encompassing theme of this symposium is "life stress and illness," and the specific research reports range from broad epidemiologic studies of patterns of manifest illness in large populations to investigations of specific biochemical and neuroendocrine changes in individual subjects. All these reports are concerned with the interplay between psychological states ("stress" states) and changes in physiological functioning (biochemical, neuroendocrine, electrophysiological). Their findings should permit refinement, to some degree, of our concepts of psychomatic interrelationships, with the new data being integrated *a posteriori* into the standing operational theoies of psychosomatic medicine.

In our studies we investigated several aspects of an individual's experience—personality, conflict and physiologic response. Recent refinements in the methodologic approach to the assessment of each of these factors have been developed. These are of two major types—the multivariate statistical analysis of data collected simultaneously from two or more domains (psychological, social-demographic, physiological, etc.), and the structuring of experiments to hold one or more domains as nearly constant across subjects as possible, thereby controlling for its effect.

The application of multivariate statistical methods[26] to behavioral data has been discussed in a number of recent articles. Fen described in general terms the usefulness of multivariate techniques for both the qualitative configuration of a case and the quantitative generalization of sample cases,[13] and others have emphasized specific types of techniques, such as multiple regression, factor analysis, cluster analysis and discriminant analysis,[10,18,24] as well as time series analysis of the single case[16] and biological rhythm analysis (rhythmometry).[27] The other broad approach, that of attempting to control for certain factors in the design of studies, has been exemplified in the studies of Navy men in situations evocative of unequivocal biochemical stress responses.

Historically, the military ambience has been viewed as one of occasional potent stressors. A constant flow of publications, ranging from anecdotal collections to research reports, attests to the kaleidoscopic array of military life situations that require extreme adaptability to hostile environments and/or the performance of complex, often tedious tasks.[1,4,5,14,19,34]

Some environmental factors that can vary to an extreme degree are the following:

1. TEMPERATURE. Aboard the same Navy ship, men in the deck divisions may be working in below-freezing weather, while the boiler-

men in the engine compartments may be in a steamy, oily environment with an ambient temperature over 100° F.[29] Men may work in these environments for eight to sixteen hour shifts. The wintering-over parties in Antarctica are exposed for months to outside temperatures as low as —50° F, whereas survival school trainees may be kept confined (for short periods) in spaces that reach 130° F.

2. INTERPERSONAL CONTACT. Prisoners of war may be isolated for many years, while men aboard ship may have only a few square feet of personal space and may hardly ever be alone. Men on two-month nuclear submarine patrols are isolated from the rest of the world but live in relatively crowded quarters.[12]

3. DEGREE OF PRIOR TRAINING. Recruits often are exposed to relatively mild changes of temperature, activity, sleep-wake cycles, etc., but they may respond with a substantial number of stress-related illnesses. Exquisitely trained astronauts, on the other hand, may respond to sudden crisis on space missions, such as the Apollo 13 flight, with complete self-control and mastery of the problem at hand.

4. ROLE RELATIONSHIPS. The individual may be a leader, having to make decisions about exposing himself and his men to dangerous encounters, or he may be a follower, dependent on someone else's judgment for his own safety.

5. PERSONAL DANGER. The life-threatening aspects of the environment may be severe, as with men in a forward fire base or aviators flying over enemy territory, or they may be of no consequence.

6. DURATION OF EXPOSURE. A challenging and threatening task may be prolonged, as with the sixteen-week Navy underwater demolition team training course, or it may be a matter of only a few seconds, as with naval aviators landing on an aircraft carrier.

In all of these environmental aspects the psychological and physical tolerance limits of normal, healthy individuals constantly are being challenged. For example, the Navy is expanding its underwater programs in terms of depth of habitats, duration of stay beneath the surface, number and complexity of job assignments, and numbers of men trained for undersea work. The occupancy of permanent undersea naval bases by considerable numbers of men is within the foreseeable future. Also, naval aviation is requiring men to master increasingly sophisticated aircraft and electronic weapon systems, and at the same time these men are being exposed to increasingly sophisticated countermeasures by hostile forces, such as surface-to-air missiles. Other military environments, too, such as antarctic stations and space stations, will require a greater adjustment to longer missions and more complex task demands.

Our definitions of stress situations and responses incorporate to some extent the theories of the early psychosomatists, such as physiological response specificity, but in addition they permit an operational definition of environmental stress with a measurable endpoint, rather than limiting researchers to an intuitive description of a particular environmental event as stressful. For example, landing jet aircraft on a carrier in the ocean intuitively would be a stressful experience, but it carries a different significance, in terms of the state of the total organism, to different men in the same aircraft. Similarly, men under the same threat of attack by enemy forces may have different states of physiologic activation depending on their perceived role in the combat situation.[4]

In recent years, a number of carefully controlled laboratory studies with experimental animals has shown that for any given hormone, different stress conditions can result in different changes in that hormone. The unidimensional concept of Selye's "general adaptation syndrome" implying that the hypothalamic-pituitary-adrenal cortical axis is the master index of physiological stress responses[21,30] has given way to an appreciation of the overall organization of diverse biochemical and endocrine systems into coordinated patterns of response to many types of stimuli. For example, Mason has shown that, in monkeys chronically adapted to restraining chairs, different stresses such as avoidance, cold, heat and hemorrhage can elicit different changes in urine 17-OHCS levels.[23] Mason also has shown that such stress responses are not limited to a single neuroendocrine axis, but rather involve a host of hormone responses which may be divided into immediate, catabolic responses and delayed, anabolic responses based on the time course of their appearance.[22] The hormones that show the immediate response are influential in promoting energy metabolism, whereas the hormones showing the delayed response are important in post-stress rebuilding of tissues and energy stores.

Another area of research enjoying great contemporary interest is the role of biogenic amine neurotransmitters in the central nervous system. Norepinephrine, dopamine and serotonin have been implicated as neurotransmitters in those areas of the brain having to do with emotions and affective states, and with neural regulation of anterior pituitary functioning. Deficiencies of one or more of these amines have been postulated as the neurochemical basis for certain psychiatric illnesses, for example, manic depressive illness and other types of depression. In the aviator study, the increase in urine MHPG levels during the stress of carrier landings suggests that heightened turnover of brain norepinephrine can occur in normal subjects during periods of increased alerting and arousal.

The current theories of neurotransmitters are unable to include possible regional brain differences in neurotransmitter activity, because the methodologies for the *in vivo* investigation of regional changes in brain neurochemistry have not yet been developed. The current theories of amine neurotransmitters must treat the brain, or at least the limbic system and brain stem areas where these amines are concentrated, as a more or less homogeneous unit. These theories cannot do justice to the rich variegations of symptomatology that are displayed by patients with diagnostically identical illnesses, or to the great interindividual differences seen in the outwardly homogeneous groups of normal Navy men undergoing identical stress circumstances.

It would seem reasonable that such homogeneous groups of normal subjects might have quite different "total brain states" when exposed to the same set of stress conditions or circumstances, and these brain states might give rise to quite different interindividual patterns of biochemical and neuroendocrine response. It is now known that specific neuroendocrine phenomena are associated with specific "total brain states," for example, the major release of growth hormone from the anterior pituitary normally occurs shortly after the slow wave (stage 3 and 4) sleep in the first few hours of the night.[28] The release of other anterior pituitary hormones, on the other hand, normally may be associated with other phases of the sleep cycle.[28]

It will be important to apply the powerful techniques of multivariate analysis not only to the data at hand but also to future refinements in psychological, neurophysiological, neuroendocrine and other biochemical methodologies. Attempts at individual metabolic "fingerprinting"[17,36] must be paralleled by multivariate methodologies directed at individual neurophysiological or brain state "fingerprinting": during waking states at all levels of arousal, as well as during all stages of sleep. Surface electroencephalogram (EEG) power spectrum analyses, depth electrode EEG recordings, more direct measurements of brain neurotransmitter metabolism, and other ways of detection of regional differences in brain neurophysiology are all potential improvements in methodology applicable to the investigation of individual biochemical and neuroendocrine responses to psychological stress.

Another feature of the understanding of psychosomatic interrelationships which is of considerable practical importance to the military is the eventual predictability of the process of psychophysiological breakdown, nonfunctioning and the development of clinically evident pathology, especially in men who are in exotic and/or hostile environments and who must be depended on for continued performance of often complex tasks. A corollary of the exotic environment is the frequent isolation of the men, so that evacuation and replacement of the disabled member of the group is obviated.

Arthur recently reviewed some of the studies that attempted to predict success in military personnel.[2] Some effective tables have been developed which will actuarially predict the odds for the global success or failure of new naval enlistees. However, no matter how much information about the individual has been added to the prediction equation, the correlation coefficient between the characteristics of the individual and the success criterion has never been greater than about $+0.4$, leaving about 84 percent of the variance unaccounted for. Although the business of prediction undoubtedly will remain a series of successive approximations for a long time to come, the increasing demands on military men for performance success makes continued attempts at refinement of prediction essential. As information gathering about psychophysiologic processes becomes more pointed, these studies hopefully will offer more useful criteria for the prediction of performance success or failure in small groups of men exposed to specific and diverse kinds of extraordinary, and stressful, circumstances.

REFERENCES

1. Appley, M.H., and Trumbull, R.: *Psychological Stress: Issues in Research.* New York, Appleton-Century-Crofts, 1967.

2. Arthur, R.J.: Success is predictable. *Milit Med, 136:*539, 1971.
3. Barron, F.: An ego-strength scale which predicts response to psychotherapy. *J Consult Psychol, 17:*327, 1953.
4. Bourne, P.G.: Urinary 17-OHCS levels in two combat situations. In Bourne, P.G. (Ed.): *The Psychology and Physiology of Stress: With Reference to Special Studies of the Vietnam War.* New York, Academic Press, 1969, p. 95.
5. ————: *Men, Stress, and Vietnam.* Boston, Little, Brown, 1970.
6. Brady, J.V.: Ulcers in "executive" monkeys. In McGough, J.L., Weinberger, N.W., and Whalen, R.E. (Eds.): *Psychobiology: The Biological Basis of Behavior.* San Francisco, Freeman, 1967, p. 189.
7. Clark, B.R., and Rubin, R.T.: New fluorometric method for the determination of cortisol in serum. *Anal Biochem, 29:*31, 1969.
8. ————, Rubin, R.T., Kales, A., and Poland, R.: Comparison of fluorometric method for urinary cortisol with modified Porter-silber method for 17-OHCS. *Clin Chim Acta, 27:*364, 1970.
9. ————, Rubin, R.T., and Poland, R.E.: Modification of new fluorometric method for serum and urine cortisol. *Biochem Med, 5:*177, 1971.
10. Cohen, J.: Prognostic factors in functional psychosis: A study in multivariate methodology. *Trans NY Acad Sci, 30:*833, 1968.
11. Davis, R.C., and Berry, F.: Gastrointestinal reactions during a noise avoidance task. *Psychol Rep, 12:*135, 1963.
12. Earls, J.H.: Human adjustment to an exotic environment. The nuclear submarine. *Arch Gen Psychiatr, 20:*117, 1969.
13. Fen, S.: The theoretical implications of multivariate analysis in the behavioral sciences. *Behav Sci, 13:*138, 1968.
14. Grinker, R.R., and Spiegel, J.: *Men Under Stress.* Philadelphia, Blakiston, 1945.
15. Gunderson, E.K.E., Arthur, R.J., and Wilkins, W.L.: A mental health survey instrument: The health opinion survey. *Milit Med, 133:*306, 1968.
16. Holtzman, W.H.: Statistical models for the study of change in the single case. In Harris, C.W. (Ed.): *Problems in Measuring Change.* Madison, University of Wisconsin Press, 1963.
17. Horning, E.C., and Horning, M.G.: Human metabolic profiles obtained by GC and GC/MS. *J Chromatogr Sci, 9:*129, 1971.
18. Jones, K.J.: Problems of grouping individuals and the methods of modality. *Behav Sci, 13:*496, 1968.
19. Levi, L. (Ed.) *Emotional Stress: Physiological and Psychological Reactions; Medical, Industrial, and Military Implications.* New York, American Elsevier, 1967.
20. Maas, J.: Personal communication.
21. Mason, J.W.: A review of psychoendocrine research on the pituitary-adrenal cortical system. *Psychosom Med, 30:*576, 1968.

22. ————: Organization of psychoendocrine mechanisms. *Psychosom Med, 30:*565, 1968.

23. ————: A reevaluation of the concept of "nonspecificity" in stress theory. *J Psychiatr Res, 8:*323, 1971.

24. Maxwell, A.E.: Multivariate statistical methods and classification problems. *Br J Psychiatr, 119:*121, 1971.

25. Miller, R.G., Rubin, R.T., Clark, B.R., Crawford, W.R., and Arthur, R.J.: The stress of aircraft carrier landings I. Corticosteroid responses in naval aviators. *Psychosom Med, 32:*581, 1970.

26. Overall, J.E., and Klett, J.: *Applied Multivariate Analysis,* New York, McGraw-Hill, 1972.

27. Reinberg, A.: Methodologic considerations for human chronobiology. *J Interdiscipl Cycle Res, 2:*1, 1971.

28. Rubin, R.T., Gouin, P.R., and Poland, R.E.: Neuroendocrine correlates of sleep stages. *Proc V Intern Congr Pharmacol,* Excerpta Medica, in press.

29. ————, Gunderson, E.K.E., and Doll, R.E.: Life stress and illness patterns in the U.S. Navy I. Environmental variables and illness onset in an attack carrier's crew. *Arch Environ Health, 19:*740, 1969.

30. ————, and Mandell, A.J.: Adrenal cortical activity in pathological emotional states: A review. *Am J Psychiatr, 123:*387, 1966.

31. ————, Miller, R.G., Arthur, R.J., and Clark, B.R.: Differential adrenocortical stress responses in naval aviators during aircraft carrier landing practice. *Psychol Rep, 26:*71, 1970.

32. ————, Miller, R.G., Clark, B.R., Poland, R.E., and Arthur, R.J.: The stress of aircraft carrier landings II. 3-methoxy-4-hydroxyphenyl-glycol excretion in naval aviators. *Psychosom Med, 32:*589, 1970.

33. ————, Rahe, R.H., Arthur, R.J., and Clark, B.R.: Adrenal cortical activity changes during underwater demolition team training. *Psychosom Med, 31:*553, 1969.

34. *Symposium on Medical Aspects of Stress in the Military Climate.* Walter Reed Army Institute of Research, Washington, D.C., 1964.

35. Taylor, J.A.: A personality scale of manifest anxiety. *J Abnorm Soc Psychol, 48:*285, 1953.

36. Williams, G.A.: Individuality of clinical biochemical patterns in preventive health maintenance. *J Occup Med, 9:*567, 1967.

≋⋀⋀⋀⋀⋀⋀⋀⋀⋀⋀⋀⋀≋

Chapter XV

SOCIAL STRESS AND ILLNESS IN INDUSTRIAL SOCIETY

WALTER L. WILKINS

IN A SYMPOSIUM on the topic of social stress and illness, it might have been hoped that fully acceptable definitions of stress and of illness would be obtained. Yet these concepts are not tidy. Levi, in his books and monographs, has been highly consistent in his holding to Hans Selye's classical concept, although in the volumes he has been editing for the WHO series, other definitions and modifications have been found. For instance, in Levi's 1971 volume, *Society, Stress, and Disease*, the report of the first of his five Stockholm conferences, Malcolm Lader says that stress occurs when stimulation raises the activity of the organism more rapidly than adaptation can lower it. David Mechanic, the medical sociologist, puts it a little differently, but with much the same intent as Lader, "...a discrepancy between the demands impinging upon a person—whether these demands be external or internal—whether challenges or goals —and the individual's potential responses to these demands."[10] This sort of definition is much more simply put by Edward Gross* in his phrase, "the failure of routine methods for managing threats."[5] These definitions move away from the strictly biochemical and psychophysiological toward the behavioral, as John Mason, the distin-

*In his discussion of the stress of work, Gross distinguishes a sort of slow stress resulting from having a career in an organization; a stress in the job itself, the difficulty involved in doing what one is expected to do; and an organization structure stress, like having a scholarly publication held up in publication because some authors are tardy.

guished endocrinologist recommended in 1971.[9]

There is another distinction, from ergonomics and engineering, which physicians and psychologists tend to overlook, but which may be very useful—one which was raised by Singleton (in this volume). Ergonomists like to limit the use of stress to the demands, the threats, the stimulations which impinge upon the organism and to prefer the term strain for the resulting efforts of the organism to adapt to the stress. In the words of the French physiologist, "To sum up: The main point is not the term 'stress' that has to be de-dramatized from its post-Selye (1959) meaning, but that stress as such is linked to strain. A stimulus constitutes a stress for a particular system if a strain ensues within that system. In other words, under some threshold, a given factor may be a stress only for those individuals in whom it results in strain."[11]

Levi, in his response to Singleton, pointed out quite correctly that in this symposium the criterion has been illness and that the ergonomists' criterion of efficiency should not be pertinent. And yet, illness is a sort of efficiency or, perhaps inefficiency. Certain illness is a mode of performance by the very fact of its being a mode of coping.

On illness, the other half of the symposium title, the participants have been even more cautious, not wishing to get into the questions of who is ill, whether illness is in some sense a role, whether illness is partially a self-defined state (or is one ill when one's peers or superiors declare it so), how the sick person's role is described —diachronically and explicitly. And when one leaves off being ill —is this state just a reversal of the sick role? Fabrega,[4] in his anthropological account of theories of disease, distinguishes three theories which he calls biologistic (the biological functions of the organism no longer work well); the behavioral (responses to social demands are curtailed or modified); and the phenomenological (changes in states of being—feelings, thoughts, impulses—are seen as discontinuous with ordinary affairs and believed to be caused by socioculturally defined agents or circumstances). And at any particular time, a person might be considered to be normal or to be ill in terms of any one or all three of these notions.

These difficulties in definition are a reminder of the loaded camel analogy, which I learned from Martin Orne, who said that it was current at Harvard when he was a resident there. You pile straw on a camel until he is forced to his knees. Now he is sick. So you take a little straw off his back. When he can struggle to his feet again, even with a terribly heavy load, he is well.

What illnesses have seemed up to now to have had a presumption of being caused by or exacerbated by or correlated with the existence of a social stress? The participants in this symposium represent a fair sample of the research work done in the testing of the validity of the psychosocial hypotheses—schizophrenia, heart disease, depression, combat exhaustion, the concentration camp syndrome with its allusions to premature senescence, and the problem of predicting the response to surgery. In addition to the illnesses represented in this volume, there is also the interesting array of data found in Levi's books. Some of these are ordinarily regarded as physical illnesses with measurable lesions and all the other signs, while others are regarded as functional illnesses. Some are serious enough to pose the threat of death, others only reduce efficiency and a sense of well-being. Both mortality and morbidity must be regarded as legitimate criteria of illness. And in the general consideration of the relation between social stresses and illnesses and accidents we certainly cannot ignore the many years of collection of clinical data. It certainly has been demonstrated, with the sort of confidence that one can place in the cumulative clinical evidence, that there does exist a linkage between the stresses found in living and disease and death.

For instance, the work one does leaves a physical mark on one's body. The little knot on the middle finger of the student resulting from his years of notetaking and writing out his assignments, the knobs on the upper part of the feet and on the knees of the surfer, the calluses of the tombstone cutter are physical stigmata of work. Occupational medicine details a whole host of effects of various sorts of work and work hazards upon physical and physiological processes—the black lung of the coal miner is a dramatic one—and insurance companies accumulate actuarial records of perils to life and limb of various occupations, from the possible alcoholism of the whisky salesman to the life changes of combat soldiers and airplane pilots.

So, everybody knows (this is a phrase connoting that it is difficult to marshal the data tidily) that the environment one is in affects one's health. In studies of shipboard health and illness, reported from our laboratory, we have noted that the temperature, humidity, space, air, task are all related in various ways to the chances a sailor has of developing symptoms of illness and to his chances of experiencing an accidental injury. While these sorts of things, in the experiments we have been doing aboard the controlled environment of a naval vessel deployed at sea, are typical of a sailor's life, they are also prototypical of the sorts of hazards found in any occupational or even familial situation, for the home is also a place where illnesses are contracted and accidental injuries occur. There is an epidemiology of illness and accident applicable to job and home.

The Acute-Chronic Continuum

The illnesses reviewed in this volume and the evidence relating to those social and physical factors which may permit the confident prediction that such illnesses may occur—and how often and how soon—include major and minor, acute and chronic, physical and mental. One conceptual framework which may allow consideration of all of these facets is that of Dodge and Martin whose analyses, while largely based on mortality data, have applications to morbidity data as well. They feel that both chronic and acute illnesses have social factors which may be regarded as causative, but that the social factors are different for these two kinds of illness. They quote Rene Dubos as follows: "Each civilization has its own kind of pestilence and can control it only by reforming itself ... just as the great epidemics of the nineteenth century were precipitated by environmental factors which favored the activities of pathogenic microorganisms, so many of the diseases characteristic of our times have their origin in some faulty factor of the modern environment."[2]

Put succinctly, the Dodge-Martin thesis is: "these diseases which are very characteristic of our times, namely the chronic diseases, are etiologically linked with excessive stress and in turn this stress is the product of specific socially structured situations inherent in the organization of modern technological societies."

These sociologists do not discuss germ theories of disease in favor of stress theories, but they attempt to delineate the situations in which germ theory or stress theory or interactions between them are likely to be found. They have constructed an acute-chronic disease continuum. Their simple model is worth having a look at,

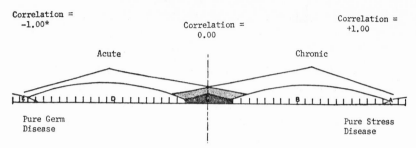

Figure XV-1. Acute-Chronic disease continuum. (Fig. 9 from Dodge and Martin.[1])

to see how some of the considerations reviewed in this volume might fit along the continuum.

Figure XV-1 shows the simple continuum. Their theory, however, involves somewhat more.

> . . . The etiological complex resulting in disease is thought of as involving three elements: the resistance or susceptibility of the host; the disease-producing agent; and the nature of the environment in which the agent and the host are brought together. This conceptual model has been most highly developed with respect to the etiology of acute, infectious diseases, but it may be applicable in the analysis of chronic diseases. In fact, it illustrates that there is not a hard and fast demarcation line between acute and chronic. It should be noted that this model lends too much emphasis to factors of an immediate nature and fails to take into consideration the time dimension—i.e. little if any provisions for the balance of accumulated effects.
>
> The basic idea behind this conceptual model is that the three elements may vary in their roles in bringing about a state of disease. Conditions may vary in the host, making him more or less capable of resisting the agent. Possible sources for this variation in the host are myriad: change in motivation, genetic constitution, aging, fatigue, personality, etc. Of particular interest to us are changes in the balance of internal stress, attitutes and physical vigor. In the case of chronic diseases we are postulating that such changes are crucial in causing disease directly—vis-à-vis the stress-disorder-disease nexus, or conditioning the host so that he is susceptible to discernible pathogenic agents.
>
> Conditions may also vary in the agent of the illness or disease. In the case of pure acute diseases the concern is with changes that make the agent—pathogenic microorganisms or viruses—virulent or weak, while

in a pure chronic disease (as conceived here) the intensity of the stress situation varies.

Of course environmental conditions within which the agent and host are brought together and interact also vary. In the case of both infectious diseases and chronic diseases we are particularly concerned with changes in the social structure and social organization and the group, community, and society which generate varying levels and prevalence of medical control; role conflict and other sociocultural patterns evocative as emotional forces; biological living conditions, food and nutrition factors, prevention and remediation practices dealing with temperature, humidity, natural disorders, etc. Obviously, the role that varying environmental conditions play in this trilogic relationship is whether the environment is such that it is favorable or unfavorable to a forceful, efficient impact of the agent on the host.[1]

At the A end of the continuum would be located diseases (and possibly deaths) resulting from excess of stress without any germ involvement. Prolonged exposure to stress would be important—as illustrated by what was called the "old sergeant's syndrome" during World War II. It is axiomatic that the longer a stress lasts, the more severe it is. In the case of the soldiers too long in the line during combat, exposed to too much noise and discomfort, too compelling a peril, the fatigue and other aspects of the stress of combat cumulated to provoke breakdown. The debate in the *New England Journal of Medicine* in 1945 over whether every man has a breaking point provides illustrations of the significance of the length and cumulative effects of combat stress. The work of Eitinger[3] and other students of the concentration camp survivors, summarized for this volume by Arthur, also shows the interactive effect of severity of stress and its duration. In a less dramatic way the work of Rahe shows how stresses in combination can add up to a critical point. The man who loses his job, is deserted by his wife, and has his house burn down encounters a cumulation of stress much more severe in their effects than if these disasters had occurred separately.

The figure suggests that the correlation at the right hand end of the chart between death rate and severity of stress would approximate +1.00. This would occur only in a situation in which no control could be exercised over the stress or its severity.

At the other end of the continuum postulated by Dodge and Martin would be diseases in which no initial amount of stress would be involved, but pathogenic organisms would be prepotent, even lethal, such as cholera. Hopefully, these are the diseases over which adequate public health measures allow some control. However, even here a cautionary admonition is in order, for it is, or used to be, axiomatic among bacteriologists that whenever they had succeeded in modifying the bodily processes so that some microorganism lost its capability of striking man low, they had also, in the process of that modification, altered the pattern of his resistances so that the likelihood of his being more susceptible to some other microorganism, which his defenses had been adequate for, increased—thus assuring not only the continued mortality of man but also the continued employment of research bacteriologists. It is suggested that the correlation between stress and death rates from such diseases at the "germ" end of the continuum would be -1.00.

It should not be assumed that there really are any diseases at the extreme ends of this scale. Because of the variety of factors mentioned in the host and in the environment, nothing that simple occurs. In every instance of a person invaded by a virus, no matter how potent, there is some stress. There may be no susceptibility narrowly defined, but there is some stress. In this volume the diseases presumed to fall under area B are those which are of most importance when we consider the social, the economic or the psychosocial factors related to disease.

In societies where the public health approaches have not been systematically applied and in which the diseases which might fall under Area D are still relatively uncontrolled, the diseases under Area B are of lesser importance. Before the widespread use of DDT, for instance, in areas which had endemic proportions of disease now controlled by such measures, it was bootless to fret about chronic diseases. It was obvious that the World Health Organization, in directing and mounting its attacks on the world's worst health scourges—those which carried off infants and children, or those which enfeebled adults so that they could not produce food and shelter—would face first the acute diseases, which should be those which preventive medicine can find a direct handle on. In the priority of things, it is inevitable, and proper, that the chronic diseases should be attacked later.

There is also the demographic principle that diseases which attack the elderly who have presumably had some opportunity to live and to contribute to the welfare of others are somewhat less urgent to conquer than those which kill off youth who have had no chance to live full lives. Thus the very proper attention to the acute before the chronic diseases.

The postulates of the Dodge-Martin theory, as it applied to those areas of illness which might be considered to be brought about by social stresses, are as follows:

1. Incidence and prevalence of chronic disease in a population varies directly with the extent of socially induced stress, which varies inversely with the stability and durability of social relationships.

2. Such stability is a function of the extent members of the population conform to the social demands of others.

3. Such conformity varies with role conflicts, which result from incompatible statuses and this, in turn, is a function of status integration.

Theorell's data, incidentally, provide new evidence of the relationship of status incongruity and myocardial infarction.

Now, what sort of people have incompatible statuses? Such factors as age and sex and race are not modifiable. They can be disguised, of course, as when younger people grow beards to appear older or older persons use various devices to appear younger. Once conceived, one's age is not subject to change—and sex and race are just about as immutable. Occupation and marital status are changeable, as are religion and some other statuses, although to change them requires some skill, or natural endowment, or effort. Change of such statuses, as suggested by Rahe's data, seems to be associated with a measurable increase in likelihood of some sort of illness. Any dramatic change of status, up or down and perhaps lateral, may be associated with modification of health status. We have noted in our research unit some examples of enlisted sailors whose academic accomplishments prior to enlistment in the Navy justified their being converted into commissioned officers. When they change their uniforms and put on their stripes, their status changes dramatically enough so that such men are transferred to a new post, where the inconsistency between their old and new statuses would be less noticed.

A drastic change in status, for the worse, can be illustrated by the phenomenon of the prisoner of war. If a pilot is shot down, he is suddenly changed from an officer with many rights and some important responsibilities to a prisoner with very few rights (and no way to enforce such rights as he may have) or responsibilities. The increase in stress can be imagined. The social context of such stress can also be illustrated by noting what changes occur in the family in such a situation. The wife of the prisoner of war is abruptly exposed to new and drastic stresses. Her concern over her husband's survival and health is accompanied by her mounting familial responsibilities by which she must become head of the household and manage children and home. Indeed any situation in which a man, as bread-winner, is severely stressed, affects the adaptation of his wife. If his job is jeopardized, her status is threatened, as a general rule. We all know exceptions, of course—giddy or simpering wives who, when disaster struck their husbands' careers by sickness or economic change, become strong, capable women; and perhaps even some who, when their husbands' careers were re-established, reverted to their earlier giddiness.

This *contagion of stress*, from husband to wife, is widely appreciated, but hardly tested in a scientific sense. Demographers have compared death rates of husbands and wives for various places and causes, but these data are difficult to interpret.

It is by no means inevitable that a person occupying a status which is in some way incompatible will be unable to cope and will suffer thereby. Some persons are tough enough or insensitive enough so that they just occupy situations which would be stressful for most of us. Such situations might be marital; we are all acquainted with married partners who seem amazingly incompatible, yet they get along in some fashion. And we all know persons who thrive on job assignments which appear to be beyond their resources.

The Social and the Biological

A basic assumption in all of this is that certain situations or jobs or locations have environmental accompaniments which affect different people in different ways, but affect the biological and the emotional experience of such people so that they become susceptible to illness or at least result in illness rates that are higher than base rates, if base rates can be reliably determined.

This leaves open a question as to whether stress is predisposing to illness or is precipitating—a sort of triggering. It is probably not a triggering agent, unless the physical stress is overwhelming, as in the case of the decompensated soldier in combat whose loss of sleep, fatigue and reaction to noise and to danger have worn down all his physical and psychological defenses. In the predisposing argument, it is presumed that the stress conditions affect the individual in some way that makes him susceptible to certain pathogenic organisms. The emotional or physical weakening of the individual reduces his resistance to certain acute diseases or perhaps does something to accelerate the disease he may have in some certain form. Or, as suggested in the discussions by Rahe and by Brown in this volume, it may foreshorten the time it takes a disease which was going to happen and bring it about days or weeks or years earlier.

As sociologists, Dodge and Martin divide the world into two camps in regard to levels and types of illness which result in mortality and thus show up in mortality tables:

1. Those parts of the world in which acute infectious and contagious diseases are common and which have high morality rates from such diseases. These will be assumed to be the so-called "underdeveloped countries."

2. Those parts of the world in which acute infectious and contagious diseases are pretty much under control, but in which mortality affects older people who suffer from chronic ailments. These would be the economically and industrially developed countries.

Implicit in their argument is the thesis that underdeveloped countries have less status ambiguity and thus less chronic disease.

This conceptual framework of Dodge and Martin should be reviewed in the light of Levi's chart. Levi has pointed out,

> The highest stress levels are usually found at the extremes of the stimulation continuum, i.e. during exposure to over- and under-stimulation. In general, deprivation or excess of almost any influence is found to be stress provoking in Selye's use of the word. For instance, high stress levels may be induced during sensory deprivation and sensory overload, in response to extreme affluence as well as to extreme poverty, parental overprotection as well as parental deprivation, extreme permissiveness as well as extreme restriction of action, etc.

In Levi's formulation, both too much and too little should be equally provocative of illness. Yet, Rahe's studies do not show that extremely low life crisis scores predict illness. And surely Paykel's data (as presented at this symposium) show that undesirable events or, George Brown would add, those perceived as undesirable, have more potency for predicting illness than do desirable ones. Paykel's work demonstrates that some events are upsetting, but not such as to provoke maladjustment; in his phaseology, entrances are better than exits and desirable events better than undesirable ones. In Rahe's events, the birth of a son may be upsetting to one's routine, but is hardly a catastrophe, but the death of a spouse is both upsetting and prodromal. Certainly within one's family, entrances are better than exits.

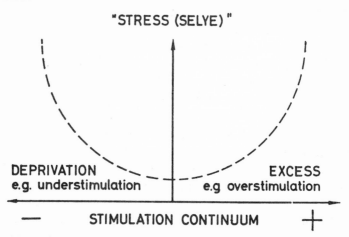

Figure XV-2. Relation between physiological stress and level of stimulation. (Fig. 1:3 from Levi.[6])

Parenthetically, it may be noted that effects of over-stimulation, the right extreme on Levi's chart (Fig. XV-2), may be noticed in aspects of maladaptation other than acute or chronic illness. Lipowski[7] of McGill has shown how a surfeit of attractive information inputs can bring about a psychological conflict and provoke coping strategies to reduce the intensity of resulting unpleasant feelings. Stimulus surfeit, he feels, has far-reaching consequences for contemporary youth and contribute to alienation and confusion.

As might be expected in a symposium devoted to such a broad topic, there are differences in the definitions of the problems. Some feel, like George Brown, that the problems define the theory to be used to explain them; others feel that theory influenced what problems were defined. All agree with Singleton's axiom that poor definition of problems leads to poor measurement of factors. The criterion emphasis in the present symposium has been on illness. Levi reminded us that effects of social stress may well be found on efficiency, economic well-being, personal happiness and even political tranquility. Illness, while by no means the only area where the effects of social stress may be assessed, is an appropriate and important criterion.

Research scientists disagree on the issue of the cumulation of stress. It is commonly assumed that a nagging wife can drive a man to drink, but we do not know how long it takes or how severe the nagging must be. It is heartening to learn, from Brown's work, that an event long in the past may have little if any effect on our present adjustment and health, and to know that Rahe agrees. Arthur's review, too, of the late adjustment of prisoners shows that childhood events may be much less powerful in adult adjustment and illness than early Freudian hypotheses had held. Nevertheless, as Arthur pointed out, events of a quarter century ago, if traumatic enough, may still have an overwhelming effect on persons who suffered the stress.

Unanswered as yet is the selection of mode of breakdown. The tables of data from Theorell and from Paykel suggest that much the same sort of stress may provoke in one man a myocardial infarct and in another a depression. Patient research may in the long run throw light on this question.

The final lesson is that constant communication between internist, endocrinologist, epidemiologist, psychiatrist, sociologist, ergonomist, psychologist, cardiologist and the others is necessary. In bringing us up to date on some developments in biochemistry, Rubin reminded us how early we become arrested in our knowledge in fields other than our own. So we must arrange for our studies to be planned, our techniques carried out, our data analyzed, and our interpretations reached with the solid cooperation of our colleagues from disciplines other than our own. Obviously this cooperation should be cross-national as well as cross-disciplinary, for it is enlightening to see how other people face their crises and stresses whether in research or in life.

REFERENCES

1. Dodge, D.L., and Martin, W.T.: *Social Stress and Illness.* Notre Dame, Ind., University of Notre Dame Press, 1970.
2. Dubos, R.: *Man Adapting.* New Haven, Conn., Yale University Press, 1965.
3. Eitinger, L.: Acute and chronic psychiatric and psychosomatic reactions in concentration camp survivors. In Levi, L. (Ed.): *Society, Stress and Disease,* Vol. I. The psychosocial environment and psychosomatic disease. London, Oxford University Press, 1971.
4. Fabrega, H., Jr.: The study of disease in relation to culture. *Behav Sci,* 17:183-203, 1972.
5. Gross, E.: Work organization and stress. In Levine, S., and Scotch, N. (Eds.): *Social Stress.* Chicago, Aldine, 1970.
6. Levi, L.: Stress and distress in response to psychosocial stimuli. *Acta Medica Scand,* Suppl. 528, 1972.
7. Lipowski, Z.J.: Surfeit of attractive information inputs: A hallmark of our environment. *Behav Sci, 16:*467-471, 1971.
8. Mason, J.W.: Strategy in psychosomatic research. *Psychosom Med,* 32:427-439, 1970.
9. ————: A re-evaluation of the concept of non-specificity in stress theory. *J Psychiatr Res, 8:*323-333, 1971.
10. Mechanic, D.: Invited commentary on self, social environment, and stress. In Appley, M.H., and Trumbull, R. (Eds.) *Psychological Stress.* New York, Appleton-Century-Crofts, 1967, pp. 199-202.
11. Parrot, J.: The measurement of stress and strain. In Singleton, W.T., Fox, J.G., and Whitfield, D. (Eds.): *Measurement of Man at Work.* London, Taylor and Francis, 1971.
12. Singleton, W.T.: Measurement of man at work with particular reference to arousal. In Singleton, W.T., Fox, J.G., and Whitfield, D. (Eds.): *Measurement of Man at Work.* London, Taylor and Francis, 1971.

AUTHOR INDEX

A

Abel, T., 197, 205
Adamson, J. D., 201, 205
Agmon, J., 92, 104
Allalouf, D., 92, 104
Ander, S., 91, 100, 101
Anderson, C. L., 201, 205
Andersson, F., 91, 101
Anthony, E. J., 189, 194
Antonowsky, A., 91, 102
Antonovsky, A., 165, 187
Appley, M. H., 5, 7, 235, 239, 242, 254
Arieti, S., 199, 205
Arlow, J. A., 90, 102
Arthur, R. J., 53, 57, 58, 60, 61, 62, 63,
65, 66, 68, 69, 70, 71, 73, 76, 77, 80, 83,
87, 88, 89, 106, 109, 114, 119, 208, 209,
211, 212, 213, 214, 215, 224, 225, 226,
227, 230, 232, 239, 240, 241
Averill, J. R., 81, 88

B

Bailey, M. A., 92, 103
Bajusz, E., 12, 17, 18, 29, 32
Barchha, R., 136, 162
Barron, F., 229, 240
Bassell, J., 83, 87
Bauer, C. B., 19, 31
Beebe, G. W., 204, 205
Benjamin, B., 91, 92, 102, 103
Bennett, L., 60, 77, 81, 88, 107, 119
Bepler, C. R., 90, 104
Bergen, T., 71, 73, 77
Berkun, M. M., 17, 29
Berry, F., 229, 240
Bettelheim, B., 197, 205
Bialek, H. M., 17, 29
Biderman, A. D., 202, 205
Biersner, R. J., 69, 70, 77, 209, 213, 215,
225

B

Birley, J. L. T., 165, 168, 171, 181, 186,
187, 188
Bittner, E., 199, 204, 207
Board, F., 18, 29
Bonami, M., 91, 102
Bourne, P. G., 83, 86, 212, 224, 232, 237,
240
Boysen, A. M., 201, 205
Bradess, V. A., 106, 120
Brady, J. V., 83, 86, 228, 240
Breslow, L., 90, 102
Brill, N. Q., 201, 204, 205
Brod, J., 100, 102
Bross, I. D. J., 208, 224
Brown, G. W., 136, 147, 162, 165, 168,
171, 173, 174n, 181, 185, 186, 187
Bruhn, J. G., 91, 102
Buell, P., 90, 102
Butcher, H. J., 35, 39
Bykov, K. M., 21, 29

C

Callagan, J. E., 202, 207
Campbell, D. T., 86
Cantrill, H., 82, 87
Caplan, G., 191, 194
Carlestam, G., 13, 29, 83, 87
Carlson, L. A., 100, 102
Carney, M. W. P., 156, 158, 162
Carstairs, G. M., 186, 187
Castelli, W. P., 105, 119
Chandler, B., 91, 102
Chapanis, A., 14, 29
Chodoff, P., 197, 199, 205, 206
Chosey, J. J., 73, 76
Clark, B. R., 83, 89, 209, 211, 212, 215,
224, 225, 226, 227, 230, 240, 241
Clayton, P., 135, 162
Cleveland, S. E., 90, 102
Cline, D. W., 73, 76

255

SUBJECT INDEX